THE LITERATURE OF
DEATH AND DYING

This is a volume in the Arno Press collection

THE LITERATURE OF DEATH AND DYING

Advisory Editor
Robert Kastenbaum

Editorial Board
Gordon Geddes
Gerald J. Gruman
Michael Andrew Simpson

See last pages of this volume
for a complete list of titles

A HISTORY OF IDEAS ABOUT THE PROLONGATION OF LIFE

GERALD J. GRUMAN

ARNO PRESS

A New York Times Company

New York / 1977

Reprint Edition 1977 by Arno Press Inc.

Copyright © 1966 by The American
    Philosophical Society

Reprinted by permission of
    The American Philosophical Society

THE LITERATURE OF DEATH AND DYING
ISBN for complete set: 0-405-09550-3
See last pages of this volume for titles.

Manufactured in the United States of America

———————◆———————

Library of Congress Cataloging in Publication Data

Gruman, Gerald J
    A history of ideas about the prolongation of life.

    (The Literature of death and dying)
    Reprint of the ed. published by American Philosophical
Society, Philadelphia, which was issued as new ser.,
v. 56, pt. 9 of Transactions of the American Philosophi-
cal Society.
    Bibliography: p.
    1. Longevity. 2. Death. I. Title. II. Series.
III. Series: American Philosophical Society, Philadel-
phia. Transactions ; new ser., v. 56, pt. 9.
[QP85.G75 1977]   081s   [179'.7]   76-19574
ISBN 0-405-09572-4

TRANSACTIONS

OF THE

AMERICAN PHILOSOPHICAL SOCIETY

HELD AT PHILADELPHIA

FOR PROMOTING USEFUL KNOWLEDGE

NEW SERIES—VOLUME 56, PART 9
1966

A HISTORY OF IDEAS ABOUT THE PROLONGATION OF LIFE

THE EVOLUTION OF PROLONGEVITY HYPOTHESES TO 1800

GERALD J. GRUMAN

Assistant Professor of History, University of Massachusetts

THE AMERICAN PHILOSOPHICAL SOCIETY

INDEPENDENCE SQUARE

PHILADELPHIA

DECEMBER, 1966

In memory of
HARRIS McKINLEY GRUMAN
1896–1952

. . . tua me, genitor, tua tristis imago saepius occurrens haec
limina tendere adegit.

Aeneid 6 : 695

This investigation was supported by research grants M-2163
and M-2686 and by research fellowship MF-10,022 from the
National Institute of Mental Health, Public Health Service.

Library of Congress Catalog
Card Number 66–25026

PREFACE

My aim has been to trace the origin and evolution of the idea of prolongevity: the belief that it is possible and desirable to extend significantly the length of life by human action. In this study, primary attention is given to developments before the end of the eighteenth century (another work, already initiated, will concentrate on events since 1800). There are, however, numerous references to modern times. As Carl Becker and Charles Beard pointed out, there is some present-mindedness in all historical writing, and I must acknowledge that this work is meant to be strongly relevant to the contemporary human situation.

I have tried to integrate, in this investigation, the history of ideas and the history of science, for a concept like prolongevity reflects almost equally the influence of philosophy, religion, science, and medicine. I have attempted also to apply some of the methods of world history, in particular, the dictum of L. S. Stavrianos that, "no European movement or institution be treated unless non-European movements or institutions of similar magnitude and world significance also be treated" (*Journal of Modern History* 31 [1959]: p. 115). Accordingly, emphasis has been given, in the earlier sections, to developments in the Chinese and the Islamic cultures so that, in a sense, this work represents an exercise in comparative history.

In covering such a vast area of time and space, it was not possible to aspire to definitive treatment. While reliance was placed, as much as possible, on primary source materials, many of them had to be used in translations from the original language. And not a few promising leads had to be abandoned, so that the over-all project could be achieved. I should appreciate it if readers and reviewers would let me know of significant omissions or variations in interpretation.

* * * *

In writing this monograph, I owe the deepest gratitude to Professor I. Bernard Cohen and Professor Crane Brinton of Harvard University for important aid and encouragement, over a number of years, in all aspects of the work. Without the generous financial support of the National Institutes of Health, it might have been impossible to complete this research project; in this regard, I want to express my appreciation to Professor Benjamin Spector, Dr. Jeanne L. Brand, and Dr. Frederic D. Zeman. As part of the policy of Lake Erie College in the encouragement of research, President Paul Weaver made available to me a grant to be used in preparing this manuscript for publication. Others whose efforts I should like to cite in connection with this scholarly venture are Professor George Rosen,

Professor Arthur Schlesinger, Jr., the late Professor Henry E. Sigerist, Dr. Edwin D. Harrington, my mother Jeanne (Gruman) Jacobson and my wife Joan.

* * * *

It may be suitable to mention here the places where material related to this study already has been presented: in 1959, lectures on Taoist prolongevitism at the Benjamin Waterhouse Medical History Society (Boston) and at the Johns Hopkins Institute for the History of Medicine; in 1960, a lecture on medical alchemy at the annual dinner of the Boston Medical Library and a paper on medical alchemy at the annual meeting of the History of Science Society; in 1961, a lecture on "The Aging Population and the Idea of Prolongevity" at the Johns Hopkins School of Public Health and a paper at the Johns Hopkins Medical History Club which appeared as "The Rise and Fall of Prolongevity Hygiene: 1558–1873" in the *Bulletin of the History of Medicine* 35 (1961): pp. 221–229; in 1963, a paper on Enlightenment prolongevitism at the annual meeting of the History of Science Society.

My studies in the general history of gerontology led to an article "An Introduction to Literature on the History of Gerontology" in the *Bulletin of the History of Medicine* 31 (1957): pp. 78–83. I initiated a resolution, approved by the Gerontological Society at its meeting of 1958, which established a Committee on the History of Gerontology; under the co-chairmen, Drs. J. T. Freeman and I. L. Webber, the first series of four papers was presented at the annual meeting of 1963.

Another category of research intimately related to this monograph is that on C. A. Stephens and his doctrine of natural salvation: articles on Stephens appeared in the *New England Journal of Medicine* 254 (1956): pp. 658–660 and in *Geriatrics* 14 (1959): pp. 332–336. Through the efforts of Louise Harris, a comprehensive collection of material on Stephens is being built up for the Special Collections Library at Brown University, and a series of books is being published.

Growing directly out of the work on Stephens were my note "Saving our Primary Source Materials" in *Isis* 48 (1957): pp. 184–185 and editorial "Preserving the Stuff of History" in *Science* 127 (1958): p. 1471 which led to the Conference on Science Manuscripts in 1960 in Washington. The credit for the organization of the Conference must go to Professor Nathan Reingold and his committee; the proceedings appeared in a special issue of *Isis* 53 (1962).

G. J. G.

Department of History
University of Massachusetts
Amherst, Mass.

A HISTORY OF IDEAS ABOUT THE PROLONGATION OF LIFE

The Evolution of Prolongevity Hypotheses to 1800

GERALD J. GRUMAN

CONTENTS

I. INTRODUCTION

Oh that there were a medicine curing age . . .
Regimen of Health of Salerno (eleventh century)[1]

THE PROBLEM OF DEATH

The problem of death is a central part of the dilemma of modern man. This concern stems largely from the fact that the modern era has been characterized by a marked decline of faith in supernatural salvation from death, i.e., immortality and resurrection by divine fiat. While these beliefs still are adhered to by many in times of bereavement, their role in everyday life has been weakened greatly, and attention has become centered on the things of this world, especially on the increasing production and distribution of goods and services. Yet, despite the material satisfactions of modern life, the individual feels hollow and powerless when faced by death. One response, and a widespread one, is to attempt to ignore the issue by placing a taboo on it.[2] Another outlook is that of neo-orthodoxy, which focuses attention on death in order to justify a theological standpoint which is essentially medieval.[3] A third approach is that of the secular existentialists, who emphasize death and the "absurdity" of the individual, so as to sharpen man's sense of moral responsibility.[4]

---

[1] *Regimen sanitatis Salernitanum,* John Harington, transl., in F. R. Packard and F. H. Garrison, eds., *The School of Salernum* (New York, 1920), p. 112.

[2] "Our own era simply denies death. . . . Thus the fear of death lives an illegitimate existence among us." Erich Fromm, *Escape from Freedom* (New York and Toronto, 1941), pp. 245–246.

[3] E.g., Reinhold Niebuhr, *Faith and History* (New York, 1951), pp. 75–78, 156–157.

[4] E.g., Jean-Paul Sartre, *Nausea,* Lloyd Alexander, transl. (Norfolk, Connecticut, 1959). Two recent books by Jacques Choron provide useful surveys of past and present concepts of death; they are *Death and Western Thought* (New York and London, 1963) and *Modern Man and Mortality* (New York, 1964). For a fine collection of recent psychological and sociological papers on attitudes towards death, see Robert Fulton, ed., *Death and Identity* (New York, London, Sydney, 1965). On literary views, see Frederick J. Hoffman, *The Mortal No: Death and the Modern Imagination* (Princeton, 1964).

To bring the modern dilemma towards a positive resolution, the best hope would seem to be a reaffirmation of meliorism, which, in regard to the problem of death, would entail a progressive lengthening of the span of life.[5] Indeed, it may be asserted that meliorism is an indispensable element in modern society, for a community based on industry, technology, and science must continue to advance or it will face disaster.[6] To cite the most relevant example: during the nineteenth century, the chief medical problem was that of infectious disease. Through the meliorist efforts of reformers in public health and researchers in medical science, infectious diseases have been brought largely under control, and, as a result, the average length of life has been increased. At the same time, however, a new problem has beeen created, that of an aging population; society is finding itself burdened with unprecedented numbers of disabled and indigent old people. Consequently, the community, of necessity, is diverting large sums to research into the nature of degenerative diseases and of old age itself. And it can be predicted that these efforts, whatever their motivation, will further increase the length of life. In the light of this experience, it can be seen that meliorism is an inherent component in the structure of a modern society, and, this being the case, it would seem wise to adopt a conscious and systematic policy of this sort rather than resort to it only in a halfhearted and intermittent manner.

In any consistent program of meliorism, the prolongation of life must have a significant place; it is unfortunate, therefore, that the subject sometimes is relegated to a limbo reserved for impractical projects or eccentric whims not quite worthy of serious scientific or philosophic consideration. One reason for this neglect is that there is, in philosophy, science, and religion, a long tradition of apologism, the belief that the prolongation of life is neither possible nor desirable; that tradition will be discussed in the next chapter. Another reason is the fact that there are few subjects which have been more misleading to the uncritical and more profitable to the unscrupulous; the exploitation of this topic by the sensational press and by medical quacks and charlatans is well known. Furthermore, the past fifty years have seen the failure of at least three

highly publicized remedies for aging: at the turn of the century, there was the fermented-milk fad; in the 'twenties, there were transplants of sex glands; and, in the 'forties, there was the cytotoxic serum advocated by Bogomoletz.[7]

The purpose of this book is to trace, to the beginning of the nineteenth century (but not without references to more recent events) the evolution of ideas about the prolongation of life, and to demonstrate that the history of this subject is a significant one. It is hoped that we may show that the major hypotheses relating to this subject, by and large, were reasonable deductions from the science and philosophy of the times, and it will be seen that the prolongation of life was an important factor in some of the principal movements in intellectual history—Taoism, alchemy and the Enlightenment, for example. Finally, it will be pointed out that the desire to lengthen life not only initiated alluring speculation but also stimulated research which led to useful discoveries.

THE IDEA OF PROLONGEVITY

In dealing with this subject, I have found it helpful to coin a new term *prolongevity,* which may be defined as the significant extension of the length of life by human action. The prefix "pro-" is used here in the sense of "forth" or "a moving forward," while longevity retains its customary meaning of "length of life." As to the belief that prolongevity is possible and desirable, one may refer to the idea of prolongevity or to prolongevitism.

There is an older word, "macrobiosis," which connotes the prolongation of life, but it is not exactly suitable for our purpose. The term was introduced by Hufeland in 1796 in connection with his famous book on the art of prolonging life, and later editions appeared under the title *Makrobiotik.*[8] The chief objection to "macrobiosis," and probably the reason why its acceptance has been so limited, is that the prefix "macro-" is much more suggestive of "large size" (as in macrocosm and macrophysics) than of "long duration." Another handicap of "macrobiosis" is that it has become identified with a particular method of prolongevity, that of hygiene, while what was wanted here was a word covering all methods.

The import of the word "prolongevity" (which I first used in 1955) seems to be grasped readily, and it has appeared in the writings of others. It has clear advantages over the alternatives: "prolongation of life" being too clumsy for frequent repetition and "macrobiosis" being too obscure. At times I have employed pro-

---

[5] While the political and economic crises of the present century have shaken the hold of absolute ideas of progress, they, by no means, have destroyed the appeal of contingent forms of the belief. On the persistence of progressist thought, see Morris Ginsberg, *The Idea of Progress: A Revaluation* (Boston, 1953) and Clarke A. Chambers, "The Belief in Progress in Twentieth-Century America," *Jour. History of Ideas* 19 (1958): pp. 197–224; Georg G. Iggers, "The Idea of Progress: a Critical Reassessment," *American Hist. Rev.* 71 (1965): pp. 16–17.

[6] An anthropological study, for example, found meliorism to be a distinguishing characteristic of modern American culture as compared with traditional Indian and Spanish-American cultures. Evon Z. Vogt and John M. Roberts, "A Study of Values," *Scientific American* 195, 1 (1956): p. 30.

[7] These developments will be investigated in my work *Death and Progress: the Rise of Secular Salvation.*

[8] Mirko D. Grmek, *On Ageing and Old Age: Basic Problems and Historic Aspects of Gerontology and Geriatrics,* Monographiae biologicae 5, 2 (Den Haag, 1958), pp. 67–68. Also on Hufeland, see later, chap. VII.

longevity as an adjective (as in "prolongevity hygiene") in addition to its use as a noun.

Advancing to a closer look at the definition of prolongevity, it should be noted that the phrase "length of life" (or the word "longevity") may refer to either of two different phenomena.[9] The number of years which the average person can expect to live is one meaning of the phrase. For example, in the United States, the average baby born in 1957 could be expected to live about seventy years,[10] and that figure of seventy years we speak of as "life expectancy."

During the course of history, life expectancy has increased greatly; advances have been particularly striking in the past century.[11] It has been estimated by certain historians that, in ancient Greece and Rome, life expectancy was only about twenty years. During the long period of fourteen centuries from the decline of the Roman Empire till the beginning of the eighteenth century there seems to have been only a very gradual improvement in life expectancy to about thirty years. By 1800, in the more advanced countries, life expectancy had reached thirty-five years, and by 1900, in England, Sweden and the United States, it was nearly fifty years. In the 1960's life expectancy in the most industrialized nations stands above seventy years.

In contrast to "life expectancy" is the concept of "life span." While life expectancy refers to the length of life of the average person, life span refers to the longevity of the most long-lived persons. Life span is the extreme limit of human longevity, the age beyond which virtually no one, however far he may be above the average, can expect to live. Statisticians estimate the life span at about one hundred ten years. Millions of average people can expect to reach the life expectancy of seventy years, but only a few unique individuals will fulfill the life span of one hundred ten years.

Unlike life expectancy, the span of life does not seem to have increased noticeably during the course of history.[12] In every era there seem to have been a few hardy individuals who lived beyond one hundred years. The average man may have died prematurely at twenty or thirty, but, then as now, a tiny quota of long-lived persons somehow managed to survive to the extreme limit of the life span. It is of importance that the two terms be clearly differentiated: there is a widespread and probably erroneous view that the length of life has been increased and will continue to increase almost automatically as a by-product of scientific and social changes. It is the virtue of Louis I. Dublin's definitions that they challenge this vague, complacent optimism by suggesting that there may be a sharp cut-off point, a discontinuity.

While it is necessary to point out this distinction between life expectancy and life span to allow one to cope with vital statistics, there is a danger of overstating Dublin's argument. The distinction between these concepts seems to have been employed in recent times to emphasize the difficulty involved in overcoming senescence; that is, they have been used in a moderately apologist framework. The nature of "old age" remains, however, too nebulous to allow the concept of an absolute life span to pass unchallenged. Suppose, for example, significant progress were made in controlling such degenerative diseases as cancer and arteriosclerosis; Dublin, working from the view of a statistician, feels this would extend life expectancy but not the life span; senescence would continue to operate unhindered and carry off vast numbers of victims in the years between ninety-five and one hundred ten. Others, however, basing themselves on experience at the autopsy table, state that they never have seen a death from pure "old age," and the implication is that the life-span phenomenon might be an artifact of the statisticians and not a never-yielding barrier.[12a]

Keeping in mind the concepts of "life expectancy" and "life span," just what constitutes a *significant* extension of the length of life? Reading through the literature of science and philosophy, we find a great diversity of views among those who accepted the possibility of lengthening human life. One man felt that we might be able to add only a few years, another believed we might live to one hundred fifty or two hundred, and a third writer saw the prospect of immortality. Are all of these views to be classified under the heading of "prolongevity"?

The group which is easiest to classify is the one we may call radical prolongevitism. These thinkers were so optimistic that they foresaw a decisive solution to the problems of death and old age; they aimed at the attainment of virtual immortality and eternal youth. Most Taoists of ancient China belong in this category as do also many of the medieval Latin alchemists. In the modern period, Condorcet supported the radical view and so did the Englishman, William Godwin, and the interesting nineteenth-century American, C. A. Stephens. All shared the belief that human life may be lengthened indefinitely, and there can be no question at all that they were proponents of "prolongevity."[13]

---

[9] Louis I. Dublin, A. J. Lotka, and M. Spiegelman, *Length of Life: a Study of the Life Table* (revised ed., New York, 1949), pp. 27–28.

[10] Louis I. Dublin, "Outlook for Longevity in the United States," *Newsletter Gerontological Society* 4, 2 (1957): p. 3.

[11] *Idem.*

[12] *Idem.*

[12a] *Cf.* the meliorist statements by Sir Charles Dodds and by Desmond King-Hele in Nigel Calder, ed., *The World in 1984* (Baltimore and Harmondsworth, 1965) 2: pp. 22–24, 188–189.

[13] On Taoism, see chap. IV and V; on alchemy, see chap. VI; on Condorcet, Godwin, and Stephens, see chap. VIII. For a perceptive, though not very sympathetic, account of radical prolongevitism in modern (mainly Russian) thought, see Peter Wiles, "On Physical Immortality," *Survey* (London) 56 (1965), pp. 125–143 and 57 (1965), pp. 142–161.

The other group of optimists might be named the moderate prolongevitists. These thinkers proposed the possibility of a limited increase in the length of life. There is much variation in the ideas of the moderates; some thought in terms of centuries, while others foresaw the extension of life by only a few years. Because of the wide range of opinion among the moderates, it is difficult sometimes to judge which of them are to be included in a study of prolongevitism. In deciding where to draw the line, it often is necessary to take into consideration the situation in science and philosophy at the time the person was writing. The Renaissance hygienist Cornaro and his followers represent a moderate form of prolongevitism.[14]

To provide perspective for what follows, a few words may be said about the present situation regarding prolongevitism. If someone writes today that life expectancy might be extended by several years, or even by five or ten years, it is hardly worth while to consider his view under the heading of "prolongevity." The average length of life has increased so strikingly during the past century that nearly anyone can foresee the possibility of a certain degree of further extension. All that is needed is something like the discovery of a more powerful drug against tuberculosis or the initiation of more effective measures to prevent automobile accidents or the extension of better medical facilities to Negro citizens, and one can envision life expectancy inching upwards. Without any radical innovation in science or philosophy, we can look forward to an increase in life expectancy beyond seventy years, gradually approaching but never reaching the life span fixed at about one hundred ten years.

It is around the concept of life span that the question of prolongevity is discussed today. The life-insurance statisticians have established so clearly the limit of one hundred ten years, that anyone foreseeing an extension of life much beyond that mark can be classified as a prolongevitist. In some cases, the figure of one hundred ten years is sharply challenged. Russian scientists, for example, claim that a number of Soviet citizens live longer, some even reaching one hundred forty-five. Most of these examples of extreme longevity occur in areas like the Caucasus where records of vital statistics are inadequate, and non-Russian scientists have been loath to accept their validity. By and large, the idea of prolongevity in recent times centers on the possibility of surpassing the one-hundred-ten-year limit by means of some scientific or medical breakthrough, particularly in regard to the problem of old age itself.

Before leaving the subject of "length of life," it should be stated that nearly all prolongevitists have had in mind not merely an increase in time *per se* but an extension of the healthy and productive period of life. It sometimes is argued in opposition to the prolongation of life, that it is better to die comparatively early rather than have to endure the disabilities of old age; an

14 On the hygienists, see chap. VII.

example of this line of thought is the Greek legend of Tithonus recounting the wretched fate of a man who was granted immortality but not eternal youth.[15] This objection, however, is founded on a misreading of the purpose of prolongevitism, which, by and large, has aimed at the "cure" of old age. The questions raised by the prolongevitists are not limited to whether longevity can be enlarged but include also: what is the nature of old age itself; is it to be considered a natural phase or a disease; is it inevitable or is it subject to amelioration? For the most part, the search for long life has gone hand in hand with the quest for rejuvenation.

The goal of prolongevity is not to lengthen the suffering and infirmity often associated with age. One finds very little of the eccentric, compulsive, counting-of-years personality in the writings of prolongevitism. The overly-competitive, sometimes-senile type who scans obituary columns in the search for a morbid feeling of superiority in outliving his contemporaries is no hero in prolongevity literature; nor is there much encouragement for the hypochondriac obsessed with health and youth. Perhaps the closest we come to egotism might be the Renaissance hygienist Cornaro, but his hygienic method was a simple one, easy to follow, and the type of old age he generously offered to make possible for all persons was seen as a happy, creative, and lovely time of life. Some of the Taoist adepts might be open to charges of narrow self-seeking: Taoist saints are pictured usually as gnarled and malformed and secretive about their methods of attaining great longevity. However, the general tone of Taoist writing and painting is benevolent and humanitarian; the successful adept, although aged in appearance, possessed powers and joys surpassing those of youth and usually his personality was good-humored and even whimsical. The type of prolongevitist most often presenting a secretive, selfish and overly-fastidious personality would be the alchemist, but here again the picture must be balanced against prejudice: the writings of a Roger Bacon offer many attractive, healthy-minded qualities; for example, he thoroughly rejected the neurotic over-elaboration of Galenic hygiene.

Having discussed longevity and what may be held to constitute a significant extension of it, we turn to the question of the means by which prolongevity is to be brought about. In the definition of prolongevity, the phrase "by human action" was chosen so as to exclude any increase in length of life induced directly by divine fiat or by large-scale natural factors not yet under human control, such as changes in climate. Despite this restriction, there still have to be considered a wide variety of methods, which may be classified as follows: "religious" prolongevitism would be that which focuses on the propitiation of supernatural powers; one form of it, the Hebrew, is mentioned later, and another,

15 On Tithonus, see chap. II, section on myth and legend.

that of the Taoists, is described in some detail.[16] A second type would be "magic" prolongevitism based on naive and primitive methods aimed at manipulating supernatural and also, to some extent, natural powers; magic prolongevitism enters our study most directly in the chapter on folklore, but it also is not far from attention in Taoism and alchemy.

Because it is hoped to produce something of value to present-day science, the emphasis in this work will be largely on *natural* prolongevitism, the sort that is founded on non-supernatural means. There are, of course, a number of different categories falling under this heading. If based on exact observation and experiment, it might be termed "scientific" prolongevitism; this, however, is too rigorous a requirement to 'be met by most of the hypotheses elaborated during the period before 1800. Somewhat less severe in its methodology, yet at the same time subject to professional discipline, would be "medical" prolongevitism, a designation which would cover some of the ideas of Descartes and Francis Bacon.[17] There also might be mentioned "hygienic" prolongevitism, as in Cornaro and his followers, and "ethical" prolongevitism, as in William Godwin; and, were we to discuss the nineteenth-century utopians, the phrase "social" prolongevitism could be added. The largest segment of this study will be concerned with *proto-scientific* prolongevitism, the term proto-science designating a stage midway between magic and science, as, for example, many theories of the Taoists and the alchemists.[18] Much of the history of prolongevity would have to be ignored if a rigid distinction were attempted between "supernatural" and "natural" means. Lynn Thorndike, in his monumental work, has demonstrated the persistence of magic into the era of early modern science, and the studies of Carl Becker have traced "medieval" religious concepts into the Enlightenment.[19]

Finally, it may be useful to make clear the distinction between two words which will appear from time to time—gerontology and geriatrics. The word *gerontology* refers to the scientific study of the phenomena of aging, the three sciences most concerned being biology, psychology, and sociology.[20] The biologists study senescence wherever it occurs, in the farthest reaches of the plant and animal kingdoms as well as in man. The primary emphasis, however, has been on human aging, and, therefore, there exists a definite, and not always

beneficial, bias in gerontology in favor of medical considerations. As to psychology and sociology, they also play an important role in gerontology; in the *Journal of Gerontology*, for example, along with papers dealing with biological studies, there always are others presenting research in psychology and sociology.[21]

In contrast with gerontology is *geriatrics,* which is concerned with the strictly medical aspects of aging.[22] While gerontology investigates aging in all plant and animal organisms, geriatrics limits itself to the problems of aged humans. If gerontology is considered the "pure" science approach to the question of aging, then geriatrics would fit into the category of "applied" science and technology. Just as pediatrics is the branch of medicine which cares for patients in the early years of life, so geriatrics is the medical specialty which treats the illnesses of elderly patients.[23]

II. APOLOGISM

Who craves excess of days,
    Scorning the common span
    Of life, I judge that man
A giddy wight who walks in folly's ways.
                    Sophocles, *Oedipus at Colonus* [1]

In order to evaluate the development of the idea of prolongevity, it is helpful first to examine some of the

---

[16] On Hebrew ideas concerning the length of life, see chap. II, section on religion. On the Taoist spiritual techniques, see chap. V.

[17] On Descartes and Bacon, see chap. VIII.

[18] The term "proto-science" is borrowed from Joseph Needham, *Science and Civilization in China* (Cambridge, 1954 ff.) 2: p. 34.

[19] Lynn Thorndike, *A History of Magic and Experimental Science* (8 v., New York, 1923–1958) and Carl Becker, *The Heavenly City of the Eighteenth-Century Philosophers* (New Haven, 1932).

[20] The word "gerontology" apparently was introduced by Metchnikoff in 1903. Élie Metchnikoff, *The Nature of Man: Studies in Optimistic Philosophy* (New York, 1903), p. 298.

[21] For an over-all survey of contemporary gerontology, see Nathan W. Shock, *Trends in Gerontology* (2nd ed., Stanford, 1957). Thought-provoking studies of the bio-medical aspect are Alex Comfort, *Ageing: The Biology of Senescence* (New York, 1964) and his less technical *The Process of Ageing* (New York, 1964). A standard work is Albert I. Lansing, ed., *Cowdry's Problems of Ageing: Biological and Medical Aspects* (3rd ed., Baltimore, 1952). For exhaustive bibliographies, see Nathan W. Shock, *A Classified Bibliography of Gerontology and Geriatrics* (Stanford, 1951), and its extensions, *Supplement One: 1949–1955* (1957) and *Supplement Two: 1956–1961* (1963).

[22] The word "geriatrics" was coined by the American physician, Ignaz L. Nascher in 1909; Grmek, *op. cit.* (see fn. 8), p. 3. On Nascher, see the sensitive study by Joseph T. Freeman in *The Gerontologist* 1 (1961): pp. 17–26.

[23] The best available monograph on the history of gerontology and geriatrics is Grmek, *op. cit.* (see fn. 8). Also valuable are four other works: Frederic D. Zeman, "Life's Later Years: Studies in the Medical History of Old Age," *Jour. Mt. Sinai Hospital* (N.Y.) 8 (1942): pp. 1161–1165; 11 (1944–1945): pp. 45–52, 97–104, 224–231, 300–307, 339–344; 12 (1945): pp. 783–791, 833–846, 890–901, 939–953; 13 (1947): pp. 241–256; 16 (1950): pp. 308–322 and 17 (1950): pp. 53–68; Johannes Steudel, "Zur Geschichte der Lehre von den Greisenkrankheiten," *Sudhoffs Archiv für Geschichte der Medizin und der Naturwissenschaften* 35 (1942): pp. 1–27; Joseph T. Freeman, "The History of Geriatrics," *Annals Medical History* 10 (1938): pp. 324–335 and Joseph T. Freeman and Irving L. Webber, eds., "Perspectives in Aging," supplement to *The Gerontologist* 5, 1: part 2 (1965). For a review of these and similar studies, see Gerald J. Gruman, "An Introduction to Literature on the History of Gerontology," *Bull. Hist. Medicine* 31 (1957): pp. 78–83 and later comments in the same journal, 32 (1958): p. 188; 34 (1960): pp. 283–285 and 38 (1964): pp. 292–293.

[1] Sophocles, *Oedipus at Colonus*, in F. Storr, transl., *Sophocles*, Loeb Classical Library (2 v., London, 1924) 1: p. 261.

opposing traditions. Every proponent of prolongevitism has had to contend with the fact that within most
systems of philosophy, science, and religion, there have
been tendencies to accept old age and death as inevitable
occurrences on this earth, and to try to provide satisfying explanations for the existence of such harsh reali-
ties.[2] These explanations engendered the belief that
senescence and death are necessary and even advantageous to the individual and to the human race, and,
consequently, that it would be unwise to attempt to
lengthen life. From the beginning, prolongevitism had
to struggle against the paralyzing influence of this conformist and passivist attitude.

In dealing with this subject, a useful word is "apologism," which may be thought of as the antonym of
"meliorism." Where meliorism implies that human
effort can and should be applied to improving the world,
apologism condemns any attempt by human action
basically to alter earthly conditions. As our concern,
in this study, is limited to one aspect of meliorism, the
prolongation of life, it follows that we shall be using
apologism in a similarly narrow sense: within the
framework of this study, apologism may be defined as
the belief that prolongevity is neither possible nor
desirable. It should be emphasized here that ethical
and esthetic factors are indispensable elements in the
definitions of prolongevitism and apologism. What is
at stake is not only a scientific problem of what is
possible but also moral and esthetic questions, matters
of value, regarding the proper and appealing direction of
human aspirations. Therefore, to be classed an apologist, it is not sufficient for someone to assert blankly that
the prolongation of life is not possible; he must, so to
speak, take the offensive and claim that, moreover, it is
not desirable.

This chapter will present selected examples of the
apologist tradition to give perspective for the analysis
of the prolongevity ideas in the following chapters.
From folklore, there will be chosen several of the more
influential myths and legends which bear on the problem
of old age. In philosophy, we shall limit ourselves to
several key phases of Greco-Roman thought. Classical
science and medicine will be represented by Aristotle,
Galen, and Avicenna. And in religion, discussion will
be centered on the Judeo-Christian tradition. These
topics should be sufficient to illustrate the essentials of
the apologist outlook, but, of course, they will be
inadequate to convey the almost innumerable forms
which apologist folklore, religion, and philosophy have
developed in all parts of the world. It may be added
that there is no intention of implying that all the persons

and institutions discussed are wholly and consistently
apologist; in some cases (Aristotle, for example) there
are strong contrary currents, but the apologist tendencies are the ones singled out for attention.

MYTH AND LEGEND
GILGAMESH

The epic of Gilgamesh, which is concerned deeply with
the problem of death, is the longest and most beautiful poem in Babylonian literature.[3] Most of the available clay tablets dealing with this poem come from about
650 B.C., but indirect evidence indicates that the origin
of the story must be traced back at least to the Sumerian
civilization of about 3000 B.C.[4]

In brief, the story is as follows[5]: Gilgamesh is a
vigorous young king who, carried away by exuberance
and arrogance, bullies his overburdened subjects. To
divert him from his tyrannical path, the gods create a
man of wild appearance and titanic strength—Enkidu.
At first, Gilgamesh and Enkidu engage in bitter combat, but after recognizing each other's power and skill
they become very close friends and together travel about
seeking fame and adventure.

After a number of Herculean exploits, the over-
confident heroes violate divine law by killing a sacred
animal and by hurling insults at a goddess. The gods
decree the death of Enkidu, who subsequently becomes
sick and passes away. To Gilgamesh the loss of his
comrade is a devastating blow, for he realizes for the
first time that he too someday will have to die.

Gilgamesh for Enkidu, his friend,
Weeps bitterly and roams over the desert.
"When I die, shall I not be like unto Enkidu?
Sorrow has entered my heart.
I am afraid of death and roam over the desert. . . ."[6]

Gilgamesh becomes obsessed with the desire to obtain the secret of immortal life and decides to consult
with Utnapishtim, the Babylonian Noah, who dwells
in a distant land. After a long and dangerous journey
on land and sea, Gilgamesh succeeds in reaching the
abode of Utnapishtim, who tells him to stay awake for
six days and seven nights. The implication of this
advice is that he who seeks victory over death first
must be able to master sleep; but Gilgamesh, exhausted
by his travels, falls asleep.

One last hope remains for Gilgamesh. According to
Utnapishtim, there is at the bottom of the sea a thorny
plant which possesses powers of rejuvenation. Gilgamesh succeeds in carrying off the plant, but on the

[2] For a survey of Western views of death, most of them
apologist in tendency, see Jacques Choron, *Death and Western
Thought* (New York and London, 1963). For a collection of
mythic material (much of it non-Western) presented with an
apologist, Jungian introduction, see Joseph L. Henderson and
Maud Oakes, eds., *The Wisdom of the Serpent: the Myths of
Death, Rebirth, and Resurrection* (New York, 1963).

[3] Alexander Heidel, *The Gilgamesh Epic and Old Testament
Parallels* (2nd ed., Chicago, 1949). See also, N. K. Sandars,
ed., *The Epic of Gilgamesh* (Baltimore and Harmondsworth,
1960).
[4] Samuel Noah Kramer, *From the Tablets of Sumer* (Indian
Hills, Colorado, 1956), pp. 214–226.
[5] Heidel, *op. cit.* (fn. 3), pp. 5–10.
[6] *Ibid.*, p. 64.

way home he sees a pool of cold water and decides to go bathing. While he is bathing, a serpent appears and eats the precious plant, thereby gaining for snakes the power of shedding their old skin and renewing their lives.[7] Gilgamesh weeps bitterly, but finally he returns home and decides to be content with his lot.

The central theme of the Gilgamesh epic, according to Heidel, is the acceptance of the harsh fact that death is inevitable.[8] Life and death are matters for the gods to decide. Even Gilgamesh, who was two-thirds god, was unable to escape death. He performed superhuman feats of all kinds, but immortality remained beyond his grasp.

> Gilgamesh, whither runnest thou?
> The life which thou seekest thou wilt not find;
> (For) when the gods created mankind,
> They allotted death to mankind,
> (But) life they retained in their keeping. . . .[9]

If the superhuman Gilgamesh was barred from eternal life, it is clear that ordinary men should avoid futile yearnings and accept fate with as good grace as possible.

Thus, at the very dawn of history, man is seen struggling with the problem of death. Two basic attitudes come to the fore—rebellion or submission, and, in this case, it was the path of submission that was deemed the correct one.

PROMETHEUS AND PANDORA

The classic account of the myth of Prometheus, one of the most strongly anti-meliorist stories, is found in two short works by Hesiod—*The Theogony* and *Works and Days*. Hesiod is believed to have lived in the eighth or ninth century B.C.[10]

In résumé the story is as follows[11]: Prometheus was a son of Iapetus, one of the Titans, the gods whose rule had been overthrown by Zeus and the Olympians; he also was the brother of Atlas (who holds up the heavens on his shoulders). While Atlas was noted for his strength, Prometheus was remarkable for his cleverness and for his sympathy with mankind.

Prometheus first offended Zeus by offering to him the sacrifice of an ox which appeared to be large and rich but turned out to consist largely of bare bones. This incident aroused the wrath of Zeus against not only Prometheus but also mankind, and, as a result, the use of fire was barred from mortal men. However, in defiance of Zeus, Prometheus managed to steal a bit of fire and carry it down to earth. Zeus now exclaimed,

> Son of Iapetus, surpassing all in cunning, you are glad that you have outwitted me and stolen fire—a great plague to you yourself and to men that shall be. But I will give men as the price for fire an evil thing in which they may all be glad of heart while they embrace their own destruction.[12]

As the instrument of his revenge, Zeus ordered the gods to create the first woman, Pandora, endowed with many charming traits to camouflage her wicked nature. Pandora brought with her a "jar" filled with all sorts of ills and evils, and when she opened the jar she initiated the bad things of this world.

> For ere this the tribes of men lived on earth remote and free from ills and hard toil and heavy sicknesses. . . . But the woman took off the great lid of the jar with her hands and . . . countless plagues wander amongst men . . . diseases come upon men continually by day and by night . . . in misery men grow old quickly.[13]

Meanwhile, Zeus punished Prometheus by having him bound tightly with cruel chains and by driving a shaft through his body. A large eagle was set upon Prometheus to feed on his liver and, to increase the agony, each night the liver grew back the same amount that the bird had consumed during the day.

The moral of the Prometheus legend as told by Hesiod is that there is "no way to escape the will of Zeus."[14] The existence of old age and death as well as many other evils is traced back to the original sin of Prometheus, whose disobedience and excessive pride provoked the wrath of Zeus. It was because of the rash conduct of Prometheus that Zeus unleashed against mankind the dread children of Night, among which were "accursed Old Age," "painful Grief" and "Death."[15] Thus Hesiod, in the apologist tradition, explained old age and death as due to the will of the gods and indicated the proper role of man as one of humility and submission.

THE AGE OF GOLD

To increase the impact of the Prometheus legend, Hesiod related the myth of the age of gold.[16] According to this story, the world had seen five epochs. First there had been the age of gold during which a happy

---

[7] For an interesting discussion of the role of the serpent in myths which explain why man must die, see James G. Frazer, *Folk-Lore in the Old Testament.* (3 v., London, 1918) 1: pp. 66–77.

[8] Heidel, *op. cit.* (see fn. 3), pp. 10–13.

[9] *Ibid.,* p. 70. Brackets are used to indicate insertions by myself into the material quoted. Additions made by others (translators, editors, etc.) have been confined by parentheses.

[10] Hugh G. Evelyn-White, transl., *Hesiod, the Homeric Hymns and Homerica,* Loeb Classical Library (London and New York, 1914), p. xxvi, and Andrew R. Burn, *The World of Hesiod,* The History of Civilization (London, 1936), p. 31.

[11] Evelyn-White, *op. cit.* (fn. 10), pp. 5–9, 117–125.

[12] *Ibid.,* p. 7.

[13] *Ibid.,* p. 9. One notices a similarity between the role of Pandora and that of Eve; i.e., the relationship between original sin (pride), sex, and death; see later, section on Augustine and Aquinas.

[14] *Idem.*

[15] Friedrich Solmsen, *Hesiod and Aeschylus,* Cornell Studies in Classical Philology 30 (Ithaca, 1949): pp. 82–83, and Norman O. Brown, transl., *Hesiod's Theogony,* Library of Liberal Arts 36 (New York, 1953): p. 59.

[16] Evelyn-White, *op. cit.* (see fn. 10), pp. 11–17. The use of metals to symbolize human qualities reminds one of alchemical thought; see later, chap. VI.

race of men lived in peace and abundance. These fortunate mortals never grew old, and, when the time came for them to die, they passed away gently "as though they were overcome with sleep." [17] They continue to exist as guardian spirits doing good to mankind.

After the age of gold came the age of silver when childhood lasted a hundred years. The silver race failed to give due reverence to the gods, and Zeus angrily ended their sway on earth and assigned them a less desirable role as spirits of the underworld. The third generation of men, the race of bronze, was endowed with such terrible strength and violence that they exterminated themselves and passed away to the dank realm of Hades. After the bronze age there was a temporary improvement with the appearance of a race of heroes or demi-gods. These were the valiant men who fought at Troy, and they now live a contented life in the islands of the blessed at the ends of the earth.

Hesiod bemoaned the fact that he was born during the fifth age, the age of iron, characterized by unceasing labor and misery. The future of the iron race is bleak indeed, for Zeus is certain to destroy it. Hesiod foresaw a constant increase in strife, envy, injustice, and deceit. People will grow old more and more quickly until even new-born babies will show the marks of old age.[18]

The myth of the age of gold is fascinating, because it seems so nearly opposite to the idea of progress. While Hesiod saw the golden age in the past, the *philosophe* and the Darwinist saw a golden age in the future. To Hesiod the existence of an evil like old age was explained in terms of the regression and decadence of mankind, and he predicted a steadily decreasing life span. To a Darwinist who believed in prolongevity, old age was a vestige of the past that would be ameliorated as mankind progressed. There is some danger, however, of exaggerating the degree of Hesiod's commitment to the idea of regression. After all, Hesiod did state that the fourth generation was better than the third, and he implied that a sixth generation might be better than the fifth.[19] However, there can be no doubt that the myth of the age of gold as recounted by Hesiod served an apologist purpose, explaining old age and death in terms of the will of the gods and the deficiencies of human nature.

TITHONUS

In a "Hymn to Aphrodite" dating from the seventh or eighth century B.C., there is related a story about the prolongation of life—the legend of Tithonus. The legend appears in the middle of another story describing an adventure of Aphrodite, and, because the relationship between the two stories is very close, both of them will be included in the following résumé: [20]

Aphrodite, the goddess of love, had such power over the other gods that she was able to beguile them into mating with mortals, an act considered demeaning. In order to curb her haughtiness, Zeus managed to inflame her with desire for Anchises, a Trojan of remarkably handsome appearance. Aphrodite arranged a rendezvous with Anchises, and, during this liaison, Aeneas was conceived, the hero who was to escape from burning Troy and flee to Italy as the founder of the Roman nation.

After the love-making, Anchises begged Aphrodite to do something to preserve his good health. At first, Aphrodite seemed sympathetic to his request, as she recounted the story of Ganymede, a handsome young Trojan who had been enrolled among the immortals by Zeus. But then she changed her mind, as she related the legend of Tithonus.

Tithonus, a Trojan, was loved by Eos, a daughter of the Titans and the personification of dawn. Eos asked Zeus that Tithonus be allowed to live forever, and Zeus granted her wish; however, Eos had forgotten to ask that Tithonus also retain his youthfulness. For a time, the lovers lived happily, but then the consequences of Eos' dreadful mistake began to appear. Tithonus' hair turned gray, and after that the burdens of old age pressed upon him one after another, until he could not so much as move his limbs. There was nothing for Eos to do but shut him away in a room where he yet lies, babbling endlessly. According to another version, Eos turned him into a grasshopper.[21]

Having told Anchises the story of Tithonus, Aphrodite remarked that she would not want him to be deathless, if he had to suffer the pathetic fate of Tithonus. At the same time she did not seem willing to obtain for him a genuine immortality, no doubt because she considered him merely a passing paramour, and a rather shameful one at that. At any rate, Anchises' request was turned down.

But, as it is, harsh old age will soon enshroud you—ruthless old age which stands someday at the side of every man, deadly, wearying, dreaded even by the gods.[22]

And Anchises was the feeble old man carried out of burning Troy by his heroic son Aeneas.

The apologist slant of the legend of Tithonus is that it is unnatural and dangerous for mortals to attempt to evade death; only the gods are naturally immortal. The story also expresses that fear of old age which so often paralyzes the human desire to prolong life. What is the use of living long, if one extends, thereby, the

---

[17] This is an early version of "natural death," cf. Cornaro (see later, chap. VII).

[18] Evelyn-White, *op. cit.* (see fn. 10), p. 17, n. 1.

[19] ". . . would that I were not among the men of the fifth generation, but either had died before or been born afterwards." *Ibid.*, p. 15.

[20] *Ibid.*, pp. 407–427.

[21] Edith Hamilton, *Mythology* (New York, 1953), p. 290.

[22] Evelyn-White, *op. cit.* (see fn. 10), p. 423. The "conquest" of death by Aeneas, described in the *Aeneid* of Vergil, and the emotional reunion with his father Anchises, is referred to in the dedication of this monograph.

hardships and infirmities of old age? The Tithonus theme not infrequently appears in literature; two well-known examples are Juvenal's tenth *Satire* (lines 188–288) and Swift's "Struldbrugs" in *Gulliver's Travels* (part 3, chapter 10).[23] More recent variations on this theme are Oscar Wilde's *The Picture of Dorian Gray* and Aldous Huxley's *After Many a Summer Dies the Swan.* So persistent is the idea that the Gerontological Society has thought it prudent to adopt for its motto "To Add Life to Years, not Just Years to Life."

ADAM AND EVE

Although scholars disagree as to the date when scribes first wrote down the Hebrew traditions about the origin of the world, a likely choice is around the middle of the ninth century B.C.[24] The Hebrew version of the fall of man has, of course, enormous significance for theology, but our purpose here will be to examine it only as an example of apologist folklore. The story (and we shall present it "straight," as though it were unfamiliar) may be reviewed briefly as follows:[25]

After God had created Adam out of dust and water and divine breath, he placed him in the garden of Eden where there were two special trees—the tree of life and the tree of the knowledge of good and evil. God warned Adam, under penalty of death, that he must not eat the fruit of the tree of the knowledge of good and evil. However, he was free to eat the fruit of all other trees, including the tree of life, the fruit of which conferred eternal life.

As a companion for man, God created, out of one of Adam's ribs, Eve, the first woman. At this point, the serpent (*cf.* the story of Gilgamesh), the shrewdest of all wild creatures, appeared on the scene and, although Eve had heard of the dangers involved, the serpent succeeded in persuading her to eat the fruit of the tree of knowledge. She also shared some of the fruit with Adam, and thus, for the first time, there came into their minds the recognition of the differences between good and evil. One of the first "evils" of which they became aware was sex, and they fashioned aprons of fig leaves to cover their sex organs. God, of course, noticed their efforts to clothe themselves, and suitable punishments were meted out. The serpent was condemned to crawl on his belly and endure the enmity of man. As to woman,

I will greatly multiply your pain in childbearing; in pain you shall bring forth children, yet your desire shall be for your husband, and he shall rule over you.

Adam was punished by being consigned to a hard life of agricultural toil, and both Adam and Eve were made subject to death,

In the sweat of your face you shall eat bread till you return to the ground, for out of it you were taken; you are dust, and to dust you shall return.

God then drove forth the unhappy Adam from the garden of Eden, "lest he put forth his hand and take also of the tree of life, and eat, and live forever."

The story of Adam and Eve illustrates several apologist lines of thought. The inferior social position of women, for example, is explained in terms of the sin committed by the first woman. It was Eve who allowed herself to be seduced by the serpent, and, therefore, Eve and all women after her have been placed in subjection to their husbands. Similarly, the pains of childbirth were explained so effectively that even in the nineteenth century the introduction of anesthesia into obstetrics met with a storm of protest based on the third chapter of the book of Genesis.[26]

As to the problem of death, Frazer, the great investigator of comparative mythology, wrote that, "the gist of the whole story of the fall appears to be an attempt to explain man's mortality, to set forth how death came into the world."[27] On the basis of his studies of primitive folklore, Frazer deduced that in its original form the Eden myth revolved entirely about the question of immortality; the tree of the knowledge of good and evil, he felt, was a later addition. The two trees in the earlier version, according to Frazer, were simply the tree of life and the tree of death. God told Adam and Eve to eat of the tree of life and to avoid the tree of death, but the serpent deceived them into choosing the wrong tree and gained for himself, as in the Gilgamesh legend, the power of rejuvenation by the periodic shedding of skin. The Eden story as reconstructed by Frazer certainly places both God and man in a more amiable light: God intends to bestow the blessing of immortal life on man, and man misses the opportunity because of an innocent error of judgment. However, the version which actually was written down traced man's fall to outright disobedience of God's command, and, burdened by these implications of guilt and sin, the story of Adam and Eve has provided a strongly apologist account of the reasons why men must die.

PHILOSOPHY
EPICUREANISM : LUCRETIUS

The doctrines first expounded by the Greek philosopher Epicurus in the fourth century B.C. found their

---

[23] In the story of the disobedient soldier interred alive inside a stone pillar (see later, chap. III, fountain theme), we are given a glimpse of immortality as a hideous fate, a moral repeated in the American movie version of *Death Takes a Holiday,* in which the suffering of a sick child cannot be ended except by restoring death to the world (the play by Walter Ferris is less outspoken but has a similar point of view). See also, Tennyson's powerful poem "Tithonus" in which Huxley found the line, "And after many a summer dies the swan."

[24] Julius A. Bewer, *The Literature of the Old Testament* (New York, 1933), p. 60.

[25] Genesis 2 and 3. The quotations are from the 1952 Revised Standard Version of the Old Testament.

[26] Eve B. Simpson, *Sir James Y. Simpson,* Famous Scots Series (Edinburgh, 1896), pp. 63–65.

[27] Frazer, *op. cit.* (see fn. 7), pp. 47–77.

most eloquent spokesman in the Roman poet Lucretius in the first century B.C. Epicurus had taught that, if men developed the right attitude about death, they would lose their fear of it and thereby be enabled to live a more tranquil and pleasant life.[28] He also had reasoned that one could be just as happy in a short life as in a long one, and, therefore, the prolongation of life was not an important matter.[29]

In Lucretius' great poem *De rerum natura* ("On the Nature of Things"), there are presented a number of Epicurean arguments in support of the theme that "death is nothing to us."[30] He emphasizes most heavily the idea that all sensation ceases at death, and that, therefore, the dead cannot suffer in any way. He also asserts that it is necessary that each generation grow old and die in order to make room for a new generation (*cf.* Malthus, see later, chap. VIII). Another consolation is the thought that death has been the fate of all men, even the greatest. It would be presumptuous for one to try to escape a fate which had overcome the "King of Kings" Darius, Scipio the conqueror of Carthage, the poet Homer, and the incomparable Epicurus himself.

Lucretius feels that there is not much point in trying to prolong life, for, no matter how long we might live, the length of our life still would remain insignificant compared with the infinite duration of time during which we shall be dead.

What is this deplorable lust of life that holds us trembling in bondage to such uncertainties and dangers? . . . By prolonging life, we cannot subtract or whittle away one jot from the duration of our death. . . . However many generations you may add to your store by living, there waits for you none the less the same eternal death.[31]

Against the desire to prolong life, Lucretius also makes use of the Epicurean concept of the "fullness of pleasure," according to which there are only a limited number of gratifications, and, once these have been experienced, it is futile to live longer.[32] Nature is pictured as saying,

Do you expect me to invent some new contrivance for your pleasure? I tell you, there is none. All things are always the same . . . there is nothing new to look forward to—

not though you should outlive all living creatures, or even though you should never die at all.[33]

The "fullness-of-pleasure" concept is a key to the understanding of Epicurean apologism. In the ancient Western world there was little appreciation of the power of man to gain control over nature.[34] Therefore, the possibility of prolonging life seldom was given serious consideration. At the same time, because the idea of progress had not yet made its appearance, philosophers viewed life as a rather dreary round of the same experiences and, therefore, called into question the desirability of prolonging life. Thus, the Epicureans asserted that there was no reason to live on to see what the future might bring. Epicureanism envisioned a moderate and rather high-minded hedonism as the most desirable way of life, but on the popular level this outlook has tended to become oversimplified as "Eat, drink and be merry, for tomorrow we die."[35]

ECLECTICISM: CICERO

Cicero, the renowned Roman statesman and man of letters of the first century B.C., was influenced by nearly all the intellectual currents of his time.[36] In his youth he inclined towards Epicureanism; as he matured he considered himself a sceptical neo-Academic; in his last years he became increasingly sympathetic to Stoicism.[37]

In his essay on senescence, Cicero, at the age of sixty-two, argued that it is not old age that is at fault but rather our attitude towards it.[38] Like a defense attorney, Cicero listed the four principal complaints against old age and rebutted each of them.[39] To the complaint by the aged that they are excluded from the important work of the world, Cicero replied that courageous old men can find a way to make themselves useful in various advisory, intellectual, and administrative functions. To the charge that senescence undermines physical strength, Cicero answered that bodily development counts for little as compared with the cultivation of mind and character. To the complaint that aging prevents the enjoyment of sensual pleasures, Cicero replied that such a loss is good riddance, because

[28] Epicurus, *Letter to Menoeceus,* in Whitney J. Oates, ed., *The Stoic and Epicurean Philosophers: the Complete Extant Writings of Epicurus, Epictetus, Lucretius and Marcus Aurelius* (New York, 1940), pp. 30–31.

[29] Norman Wentworth DeWitt, *Epicurus and his Philosophy* (Minneapolis, 1954), pp. 230–232.

[30] Lucretius, *De rerum natura,* book 3, lines 830–1094.

[31] *Ibid.,* lines 1076 ff., in Ronald E. Latham, transl., *Lucretius, On the Nature of the Universe* (Harmondsworth, Middlesex, 1951), p. 129.

[32] De Witt, *op. cit.* (see fn. 29), pp. 230–232. The "fullness-of-pleasure" theme, in a neo-Stoic form, appealed somewhat to Carl Becker who presented it as a possible alternative to meliorism; see *The Heavenly City of the Eighteenth-Century Philosophers* (New Haven, 1932), pp. 124–125, 168.

[33] Lucretius, *op. cit.* (see fn. 30), book 3, lines 931–949, in Latham, *op. cit.* (see fn. 31), pp. 124–125.

[34] M. L. Clarke, *The Roman Mind: Studies in the History of Thought from Cicero to Marcus Aurelius* (London, 1956), p. 41.

[35] This theme already appears in the Gilgamesh epic, "Thou, O Gilgamesh, let thy belly be full; day and night be thou merry," etc. Heidel, *op. cit.* (see fn. 3), p. 70.

[36] Clarke, *op. cit.* (see fn. 34), pp. 56–64.

[37] Eduard Zeller, *Outlines of the History of Greek Philosophy,* International Library of Psychology, Philosophy and Scientific Method (13th ed., London and New York, 1931), pp. 255–256.

[38] Cicero, *De senectute,* Andrew P. Peabody, transl. (Boston, 1887), p. 6. *Cf.* Roger Bacon's indictment of old age, see later (chap. VI) and Cornaro's glorification of old age, see later (chap. VII).

[39] *Ibid.,* pp. 12–63.

it allows the aged to concentrate on the promotion of reason and virtue. Finally, to the charge that old age brings with it increased anxiety about death, Cicero answered along Platonist lines that death should be considered a blessing, because it frees the immortal soul from its bodily prison on this imperfect earth. Even if the soul were not immortal, he adds, it is desirable that the duration of life be limited just as a play is limited in length—an argument similar to the Epicurean concept of the "fullness of pleasure."

Cicero, reflecting the chief systems of ancient philosophy, felt that the course of the wise man is to submit humbly to the dictates of Nature; indeed, one of the chief purposes of philosophy is to allow man to pass through the vicissitudes of life with a tranquil mind.[40] Such an apologist point of view led to ready acceptance of old age and death, and, at the same time, it made the prolongation of life seem undesirable.

> Indeed were any god to grant that from my present age I might go back to boyhood, or become a crying child in the cradle, I should steadfastly refuse; nor would I be willing, as from a finished race, to be summoned back from the goal to the starting-point. For what advantage is there in life?[41]

STOICISM: MARCUS AURELIUS

Stoicism, founded by Zeno in Greece in the fourth century B.C., later spread to Rome where it attained a dominant position.[42] From the middle of the first century after Christ until far into the second half of the second century, Stoicism was virtually the official philosophy of the Roman Empire. The emperor Marcus Aurelius, who ruled from 161 to 180, was the last important Roman Stoic.

The Stoics insisted that man must learn to submit himself to the course of nature; it is not death which is evil but rather our fear of it.[43] If one cultivates the right attitude, he will recognize that death is a necessity to which he must resign himself.

In his *Meditations*, Marcus Aurelius elaborated on this Stoic point of view.[44] He wrote that one must learn to be utterly unafraid of death; in fact, death ought to be considered good, because it is natural, and because it is necessary for the proper functioning of the universe. Marcus Aurelius emphasized the impotence of man and praised the virtues of patience and humility. He argued that we should think often about death and, thereby, learn to despise the body.

Thou art even now in the throes of death; despise therefore the flesh. It is but a little blood, a few bones, a paltry net woven from nerves and veins and arteries.[45]

Again and again he returned to the theme that length of life is a matter of no importance.

> Though thou shouldst be going to live three thousand years, and as many times ten thousand years, still remember that no man loses any other life than this which he now lives. . . . The longest and shortest are thus brought to the same . . . all things from eternity are of like forms and come round in a circle . . . it makes no difference whether a man shall see the same things during a hundred years or two hundred, or an infinite time.[46]

Thus, the Stoics developed an apologist line of reasoning which excluded not only the possibility of the prolongation of life but its desirability as well.

BIOLOGY AND MEDICINE

ARISTOTLE

There is no need to mention the enormous philosophical influence of Aristotle; less familiar, however, is the fact that he was one of the greatest biologists of all time.[47] As a biologist, Aristotle investigated an almost encyclopedic range of problems, and one of those problems was the nature of old age. The core of Aristotle's work on old age is found in his essays *On Longevity, On Youth and Age, On Life and Death,* and *On Respiration,* but other relevant material appears in nearly all his scientific writings.[48]

According to Aristotle, the phenomena of old age can be understood if one assumes the aged body to be abnormally cold and dry.[49] Such an explanation of old age was not a novel one. Among the writings of the Hippocratic physicians of the fifth century B.C., there appears a scheme of physiology based on four "humors" and four qualities.[50] Thus, blood was hot and moist, yellow bile was hot and dry, black bile was cold and dry, and phlegm was cold and moist. The most interesting aspect of the Hippocratic system, for our purpose, is the way the span of life was divided into four ages with corresponding qualities: childhood (hot and moist), youth (hot and dry), adulthood (cold and dry), and old age (cold and moist).[51] Ancient

---

[40] *Ibid.,* pp. 3, 5. Peace of mind was the major goal in Hellenistic Epicureanism and Stoicism.

[41] *Ibid.,* p. 61.

[42] E. Zeller, *The Stoics, Epicureans and Sceptics* (London, 1880), pp. 36–40, and Clarke, *op. cit.* (see fn. 34), pp. 124, 133.

[43] Zeller, *op. cit.* (see fn. 42), pp. 332–334, and Arrian, *Discourses of Epictetus,* book 1, chap. 27 and book 2, chap. 1, in Oates, *op. cit.* (see fn. 28), pp. 271, 282.

[44] Marcus Aurelius, *Meditations,* book 2, nos. 11, 12 and 17; book 3, no. 7; book 4, no. 48; book 5, nos. 24 and 33; book 6, no. 49; book 9, nos. 3 and 33; book 12, nos. 23, 32, 35 and 36.

[45] *Ibid.,* book 2, no. 2, in John Jackson, transl., *The Thoughts of Marcus Aurelius Antoninus,* The World's Classics (London, 1948), p. 12.

[46] *Ibid.,* book 2, no. 14, in Oates, *op. cit.* (see fn. 28), p. 500.

[47] Charles Singer, *A History of Biology* (revised ed., New York, 1950), pp. 14–44.

[48] Aristotle, *De longitudine et brevitate vitae, De iuventute et senectute, De vita et morte, De respiratione,* G. R. T. Ross, transl., in *The Parva Naturalia* in vol. 3 of W. D. Ross and J. A. Smith, eds., *The Works of Aristotle, Translated into English* (12 v., Oxford, 1908–1952).

[49] *Ibid.,* pp. 466a–466b.

[50] Hippocrates, *Nature of Man,* parts 1–4 in W. H. S. Jones and E. T. Withington, transl., *Hippocrates,* Loeb Classical Library (4 v., London and New York, 1923–1931) 4: pp. 3–13.

[51] Hippocrates, *Regimen I,* part 33 in Jones and Withington, *op. cit.* (see fn. 50) 4: pp. 279–281.

and medieval attempts to explain old age were dominated by these traditional concepts of the four humors, the four qualities, and the four ages. There always was some uncertainty as to whether old age was cold and *moist* (as the Hippocratics had it) or cold and *dry* (as Aristotle stated), but that question need not concern us here. Both Galen and Avicenna followed Aristotle's lead, so it will be convenient for us to refer to this type of explanation of old age as the cold-dry hypothesis.

There is no inherent reason why the cold-dry hypothesis should engender an apologist attitude towards old age. However, Aristotle's explanation of old age was only a small facet of his cosmological system, a system with implicit apologist tendencies. Aristotle's cosmology strongly stresses the difference between the earth and the heavens.[52] Things on the earth are composed of the four ordinary elements: earth, air, fire, and water. Things in the heavens (the sun, planets, and stars) are formed of a unique fifth element, the "ether." Things on the earth by their very nature are subject to constant change, coming into being and passing away, generation and decay. Things in the heavens, being composed of ether, are immortal and unchanging. The mixing of the four elements in earthly organisms makes death inevitable.

Opposites destroy each other . . . it is impossible that anything containing matter should not have in any sense an opposite. . . . Hence all things on earth are at all times in a state of transition and are coming into being and passing away . . . never are they eternal when they contain contrary qualities.[53]

It follows that "what has been born must grow, reach maturity and decay." [54]

Aristotle's science was static and apologist rather than dynamic and meliorist. He neglected the study of "efficient causes," the dynamic mechanisms of natural phenomena.[55] Instead, he concentrated on "formal causes," static description and classification. He also emphasized "final causes," the attempt to understand the phenomena of nature in terms of purpose. Aristotle shunned an attitude of rebelliousness toward nature and, instead, guided himself by the precept that nature does everything for the best.[56] The conservative facets of his thought are illustrated by his assumptions that certain men are naturally destined to be slaves, and that women are by nature inferior to men.[57] Another

example of these tendencies is his expression of admiration for the ingenuity of nature to have arranged that the teeth fail in old age, when they no longer are needed because of the imminence of death.[58] To Aristotle, old age and death were natural and inevitable phenomena to be contemplated and described within a framework of moderately apologist teleology.

GALEN

The works of Galen, the physician of the second century, represent the culmination of Greco-Roman medicine.[59] Galen, who was born in Greek Asia Minor, achieved an eminent position at Rome, where he served as physician to the Stoic emperor Marcus Aurelius. But his greatest influence was to come after his death, when his writings attained a position of unchallenged authority. During the Middle Ages, when Aristotle became known as the prince of philosophers, Galen similarly was revered as the prince of physicians.

The most complete presentation of Galen's gerontology appears in his book on hygiene, in which he presents a variant of the traditional cold-dry hypothesis.[60] According to Galen, aging may be said to begin at the very conception of the organism. In the embryo the heat contributed by the male semen acts by means of a drying process on the amorphous material contributed by the female. Because of this drying, the tissues and organs are formed as the body grows and develops. However, there comes a time in early adulthood when the balance shifts, and the drying ceases to be beneficent and becomes malignant. That is when the fuel of the body, the "innate moisture," begins to dry up, and, as a result, the body becomes more and more cold.[61]

There is no obvious reason why Galen's theory of aging should exclude the possibility of prolongevity. In fact, it implied that one might live forever if the moistness of the body could be preserved; Galen, however, believed the drying process to be inevitable.[62] He limited himself to cautious hygienic measures designed to moderate, but not basically to alter, the inexorable development of the constitutional imbalance of old age.[63]

Galen's general framework of thought had several

[52] Zeller, *op. cit.* (see fn. 37), pp. 180–182.
[53] Aristotle, *op. cit.* (see fn. 48), p. 465b.
[54] Aristotle, *De anima*, J. A. Smith, transl., in Ross and Smith, *op. cit.* (see fn. 48) 3: p. 434a.
[55] S. F. Mason, *Main Currents of Scientific Thought*, The Life of Science Library (New York, 1953), p. 29.
[56] E.g., Aristotle, *op. cit.* (see fn. 48), p. 469a.
[57] William L. Westermann, *The Slave Systems of Greek and Roman Antiquity*, Mem. Amer. Philos. Soc. **40** (Philadelphia, 1955): p. 26, and Aristotle, *De generatione animalium*, Arthur Platt, transl., in Ross and Smith, *op. cit.* (see fn. 48) **5**: p. 732a.

[58] Aristotle, *op. cit.* (see fn. 57), p. 745a.
[59] The best biography is George Sarton, *Galen of Pergamon*, Logan Clendening Lectures on the History and Philosophy of Medicine 3 (Lawrence, Kansas, 1954).
[60] Robert Montraville Green, transl., *Galen's Hygiene: De sanitate tuenda* (Springfield, Illinois, 1951), pp. 6–7, 37, 195–204, 216–219.
[61] This explanation of the cause of cooling does not appear explicitly in Galen's book on hygiene but is taken from Avicenna, who attributed it to Galen. See O. C. Gruner, *A Treatise on the Canon of Medicine of Avicenna, Incorporating a Translation of the First Book* (London, 1930), p. 70.
[62] Green, *op. cit.* (see fn. 60), p. 244.
[63] For Roger Bacon's sharp criticism of this Galenic hygiene, see later, chap. VI.

apologist tendencies. Like Aristotle, he stressed the awesome contrast between earthly mortality and celestial immortality.

. . . do not rashly expect that from menstrual blood and semen an immortal animal can be produced, as serene, as ever-moving, as bright, or as fair as the sun. . . . But the ancients who were familiar with nature held that the animal itself was, so to speak, a little universe. . . . Show me then, says someone, the sun in an animal's body. What is that you ask? Would you have the sun generated from a septic and filthy substance like blood? You are mad, poor wretch! This, and not abstention from sacrifice or incense-burning, is true impiety.[64]

Galen's writings are dominated by teleological arguments which emphasize that nature always acts for the best.[65] To the question whether old age is a disease, Galen replied that it is not a disease, because it is not contrary to nature.[66] The apologist implications in Galen's thought inescapably follow from these two assumptions—that nature does everything for the best and that old age is not contrary to nature.

AVICENNA

Ibn Sina, known to the West as Avicenna, was born in Bukhara in Central Asia in 980 and spent most of his life in Persia.[67] Not only was he one of the great Arabic philosophers, but he also was, with Al-Razi, one of the two most influential Arabic physicians. In Latin Europe during the late Middle Ages, he ranked with Galen as a pre-eminent medical authority.[68]

Avicenna devoted the first of the five books of his *Canon of Medicine* to the consideration of "general matters relative to the science of medicine," and one of these matters was the problem of old age.[69] Avicenna's explanation of senescence was patterned on that of Galen. A drying process begins in the embryo and continues as a beneficial influence until the end of the period of growth and development about the age of thirty. The lamp analogy explains the decline of the body which begins at that time. The "innate moisture" is the fuel of the body, and, like the oil of a lamp,

it feeds the flame, the "innate heat." As the innate moisture dries up, the innate heat decreases, and, thus, the aging body becomes cold and dry.

Like Galen, Avicenna took a pessimistic view of the ability of medicine to block the decline of the aging body. He declared that senescence is an inevitable concomitant of life, and he ruled out prolongevity as a legitimate medical goal.

. . . the art of maintaining the health is not the art of averting death . . . or of securing the utmost longevity possible to the human being . . . every person has his own term of life . . . the art of maintaining health consists in guiding the body to its natural span of life. . . .[70]

RELIGION

THE OLD TESTAMENT

At the very beginning of the Old Testament, the story of Adam and Eve teaches that God has placed certain restrictions on the use of human power, and that it is folly for man to rebel.[71] Again, in the story of the tower of Babel, God is pictured as intervening quickly to safeguard his universal dominion against a challenge from presumptuous man.[72] Clearly, the proper role of mankind, is to "walk humbly" in the path indicated by divine law and to give due recognition to the limitations of human power.[73]

. . . the patient in spirit is better than the proud in spirit. . . . Consider the work of God; who can make straight what he has made crooked?[74]

The desirability of long life is recognized in the Old Testament, and often the prolongation of life is cited as an important reward of righteousness.[75] Such matters, however, remain completely in divine hands. It is God who decreed that man must die as a punishment for original sin. It is God who holds sway over health and disease.[76] And it is God who establishes a suitable length for the life of man.

. . . his days are determined, and the number of his months is with thee, and thou has appointed his bounds that he cannot pass. . . .[77]

There is a great deal of uncertainty in the Old Testament regarding salvation. The opinions of "the Preacher," that all is vanity, and that there is never anything new under the sun, contrast strikingly with Isaiah's apocalyptic vision of "the new heaven and the new earth" where men will live so long that one who dies at the age of a hundred will be considered a mere child.[78] The hopes of some, that God will rescue man

[64] Galen, *On the Utility of Parts*, book 3, chap. 10 in Arthur J. Brock, *Greek Medicine, Being Extracts Illustrative of Medical Writers from Hippocrates to Galen*, Library of Greek Thought (London, Toronto and New York, 1929), pp. 154–156. This passage makes a striking contrast with the efforts of the late-medieval Latin alchemists to isolate a quintessence; see later, chap. VI. The reference to "menstrual blood" reflects the ancient belief that this represented the female's contribution to conception.

[65] *Ibid.*, p. 154. Also Galen, *On the Natural Faculties*, Arthur J. Brock, transl., Loeb Classical Library (London and New York, 1916), p. 61 and *passim*.

[66] Green, *op. cit.* (see fn. 60), pp. 15–17.

[67] For biography see A. J. Arberry, "Avicenna: his Life and Times" in G. M. Wickens, ed., *Avicenna: Scientist and Philosopher, a Millenary Symposium* (London, 1952), pp. 9–29.

[68] DeLacy O'Leary, *Arabic Thought and its Place in History*, Trubner's Oriental Series (London and New York, 1922), p. 174.

[69] Gruner, *op. cit.* (see fn. 61), pp. 68–74, 360.

[70] *Ibid.*, p. 361.

[71] See earlier, section on myths and legends.

[72] Genesis 11: 1–9.

[73] Micah 6: 8.

[74] Ecclesiastes 7: 8, 13. Quotations are from the Revised Standard Version of 1952.

[75] E.g., Deuteronomy 6: 2 and Psalms 91: 16.

[76] E.g., Exodus 15: 26, Psalms 38: 1–8 and 103: 1–5.

[77] Job 14: 5.

[78] Ecclesiastes 1 and Isaiah 65: 17, 20.

from the grave, differ markedly from the despair of others who see no chance for man to escape death.[79] Without any clear belief in human progress, and lacking a compelling scheme of supernatural salvation, the ancient Hebrews sometimes gave way to severe pessimism.

> Thou dost sweep men away; they are like a dream,
>   like grass which is renewed in the morning;
> in the morning it flourishes and is renewed;
>   in the evening it fades and withers. . . .
> The years of our life are threescore and ten,
>   or even by reason of strength fourscore;
> yet their span is but toil and trouble;
>   they are soon gone, and we fly away.[80]

Some of these problems of ancient Judaism are brought to the fore in the story of Job, the righteous man who feels that he has been afflicted unfairly with the ills and misfortunes of the world. After a series of beautiful and moving passages in which Job laments the condition of man, the Lord appears and states very forcefully the immense disparity between the puniness of man and the omnipotence of God. Job then confesses his utter insignificance and repents in dust and ashes.

> And after this Job lived a hundred and forty years, and saw his son, and his sons' sons, four generations. And Job died, an old man, and full of days.[81]

The story of Job illustrates the Old Testament position regarding long life, not as something to be attained by man's power over nature, but as a divine reward for man's humble submission to supernatural authority.

THE NEW TESTAMENT

In comparison with the Old Testament, the New Testament is much more certain of supernatural salvation, much more other-worldly, and much less concerned about the length of man's life on earth. The strong faith that God will resurrect the righteous is set forth again and again, perhaps most forcefully in Paul's first letter to the Corinthians.[82] With faith focused on heaven, the things of this world seemed of little importance—a theme stressed repeatedly in the New Testament.[83] Similarly, the body was of little significance compared to the soul.[84]

> . . . we know that while we are at home in the body we are away from the Lord . . . and we would rather be away from the body and at home with the Lord.[85]

In this pattern of thought, the prolongation of life became a matter of utter indifference, and long life

on earth never was mentioned as a reward of the righteous.[86]

Death still was considered, as in the Old Testament, to be the result of Adam's original sin, but the sacrifice of Christ was regarded as atoning for the sinfulness of man and making possible the salvation of the righteous from death.[87] The Christian victory over death, however, is not immediate and direct. It still is necessary for man to die, so that on the day of resurrection he may be transformed into a higher type of being. Just as the "dead" seed is thrown into the earth so that a tree may be produced, similarly man must die so that his mortal physical body may be transmuted to one which is spiritual and immortal.[88] Thus, death not only may be viewed as necessary but also may be considered desirable. Paul, for example, meditated:

> For me to live is Christ, and to die is gain. If it is to be life in the flesh, that means fruitful labor for me. Yet which I shall choose I cannot tell. I am hard pressed between the two. My desire is to depart and be with Christ, for that is far better.[89]

AUGUSTINE AND THOMAS AQUINAS

In the works of St. Augustine and St. Thomas Aquinas, the two pre-eminent Latin medieval theologians, there appear detailed commentaries on some of the Biblical themes mentioned above. The nature of original sin, for example, was analyzed, and it was found to be essentially a sin of pride.[90] By pride was meant the tendency of man to rely on himself without regard to God and to try to raise himself by his own resources to a superhuman or godlike condition.[91] This commendation of humility and obedience was in the apologist tradition, and tended to undermine the kind of Promethean defiance which characterizes many of the proponents of prolongevity.

Thomas Aquinas' explanation of death is especially interesting, because it blended two different traditions, the Aristotelian and the Christian.[92] St. Thomas considered death to be both natural (Aristotelian) and penal (Christian). According to St. Thomas, even when Adam was in a state of innocence, his body was subject to the inevitable process of natural death described by Aristotle; i.e., the elements in the body have opposite qualities which clash and destroy each other. God, however, as a gift of grace, had conferred on Adam's soul a supernatural power which enabled him

---

[79] E.g., Job 19: 25–27 and Psalms 49: 15 contrast with Ecclesiastes 3: 19–21 and 9: 4–10.
[80] Psalms 90: 5–6, 10.
[81] Job 42: 16–17.
[82] I Corinthians 15.
[83] E.g., Matthew 6: 19–21 and 25–33 and Hebrews 11: 13–16.
[84] E.g., Romans 7: 24, 8: 5 ff.
[85] II Corinthians 5: 6–8. Quotations are from the Revised Standard Version of 1946.

[86] An exception is Ephesians 6: 1–3, but this is a quotation from the Old Testament.
[87] Romans 5: 12–21.
[88] I Corinthians 15: 35–55. Cf. the Taoist "deliverance of the corpse," see chap. V.
[89] Philippians 1: 21–23.
[90] Thomas Aquinas, Summa theologica 2: 2, question 163, article 1.
[91] Augustine, The City of God, book 14, section 13.
[92] Thomas Aquinas, Summa theologica 1: 3, question 97, article 1 and 2: 2, question 164, article 1.

to keep in check the deteriorative course of natural death. After original sin, the situation changed decisively. God penalized Adam by withdrawing the supernatural power from Adam's soul, and consequently the process of natural decay was able to cause old age and death.

One should notice that death, according to Aquinas, resulted from the body's escape from the control of the mind, and that the reassertion of rule by the mind would produce perfect health and immortality. Here, it required divine intervention to restore the hegemony of the mind, but in later times a secularized version of this mind-over-body type of immortality appears in the ideas of some of the proponents of prolongevity, for example, William Godwin and George Bernard Shaw.[93]

Also interesting is the belief that, along with death, the rebellion of the body against the soul produced sexual lust.[94] This correlation of sex and death runs through the entire history of thought about longevity. Aristotle already had described salacious males as short-lived, while in China related ideas led to the elaborate Taoist sexual techniques designed to augment and conserve the body's "essence."[95]

One of the most significant sections in Augustine's City of God is his attack on the cyclical theory of history.[96] As Bury pointed out, Augustine presented two Christian ideas which helped to prepare the way for the idea of progress.[97] First, there is the concept that history is not a circle but rather a process which had a beginning and will have an end. Second, there is the belief that history is meaningful. To these two ideas may be added a third which is especially relevant to the study of prolongevity—the belief that the purpose of history involved the salvation of man from death. In the words of the apostle Paul, "The last enemy to be destroyed is death."[98] Thus, although much of Christian thought must be considered part of the apologist tradition, it also contained elements which were to appear in the idea of progress, the idea of prolongevity and the idea of natural salvation.[99]

CONCLUSION

Apologism may be summarized within the following six major themes:

1. Prolongevity is ruled out by inherent defects in human nature: Here we have a point of view arguing

that humans lack the ability and self-control to attain prolongevity and to use it wisely. Involved here are errors of rashness, lust for power or sexual fulfillment, forgetfulness, indiscretion, and other failings which are not necessarily sinful. Some examples are the inability of Gilgamesh to overcome sleep, the carelessness of Gilgamesh which enabled a serpent to steal the plant of life, and the rash and lustful action of man in welcoming Pandora.

2. Prolongevity is a violation of the natural order: Whereas in theme one we dealt with human nature (the microcosm) and its defects, we now are concerned with the larger world (the macrocosm) and its order, assumed to be a correct and impressive one. The most cogent example is the cosmology of Aristotle, later adapted to Islam by Avicenna and to Christianity by Thomas Aquinas.

3. Prolongevity violates the divine order: This category centers explicitly on longevity. It clearly and directly refers to a supernatural and not a natural order. An example is provided by the statement in Job, "his days are determined and the number of his months is with thee, and thou hast appointed his bounds that he cannot pass." Also very influential is the passage in Psalms, "the years of our life are three score and ten"; and in the Epic of Gilgamesh we read that "when the gods created mankind, they allotted death to mankind."

4. Prolongevity is ruled out by original sin: In this grouping there is a stress on guilty conduct, especially pride, as the cause of old age and death. The most familiar version is the story of Adam and Eve as interpreted by Augustine and Aquinas. Somewhat similar are the arrogance of Gilgamesh and Enkidu in breaking divine ordinances and the irreverence of the men of Hesiod's silver age.

5. Prolongevity is of itself undesirable: This theme might be presented as a logical conclusion of any of the previous ones; however, the words "of itself" are meant to convey a condemnation of longer life on less contingent grounds. Thus, we have the story of Tithonus describing the most dreaded characteristics of old age; similar cautions are issued by Juvenal, Swift, Oscar Wilde, and Aldous Huxley.

6. Old age and death are desirable: Carrying further some of the above beliefs brings us to this theme; the New Testament, for example, viewing death as an essential step in the transmutation of humans to a higher form ("to die is gain"), a concept related to Cicero's idea of death as the "goal" of life (liberation of the soul from its bodily prison). Another illustration of this theme is the claim by Lucretius that aging and death are necessary to prevent overpopulation, a forerunner of the Malthusian hypothesis (see later, chap. VIII).

It is essential to reiterate that the examples of apologism cited in this chapter are not necessarily representative of the overall ideologies from which they are drawn. There are, in the world views dealt with (e.g.,

[93] On Godwin, see later, chap. VIII; on Shaw's ideas, see Back to Methuselah.

[94] Augustine, The City of God, book 13, section 13, and book 14, sections 16–26. The correlation of sexual indulgence and aging also appears in the writings of Godwin and Shaw.

[95] Aristotle, op. cit. (see fn. 48), p. 466b. On Taoist sexual practices, see later, chap. V.

[96] Augustine, The City of God, book 12, sections 13–17.

[97] J. B. Bury, The Idea of Progress (New York, 1932), pp. 20–23.

[98] I Corinthians 15: 26.

[99] See later, introduction to chap. VIII.

Greek mythology, Epicureanism, Aristotelianism, and Thomism), also currents favorable to ideas of prolongevity.

One of the puzzling characteristics of apologism is the strong emotion attached to this line of thought. For some reason, once a person decides that prolongevity is not possible, he proceeds to the (unnecessary) further assumption that prolongevity is not desirable. It is noteworthy how seldom the simple statement appears that, as of the present time, old age and death cannot be overcome; nearly always, the remark is found in a context of apologism. A statement of fact is made the core of a meshwork of ethical and esthetic judgments which obscure the original decision.

Some psychologists and psychiatrists find that death is not of much concern to "normal," "well-adjusted" individuals.[100] However, it also seems that the basic mental crisis concerning death occurs about the age of five, and that somehow the problem disappears from consciousness between the ages of nine and twelve, probably because our culture applies strong pressures against the expression of anger or fear about death.[101] Of some pertinence is the concept of "cognitive dissonance," the psychological finding that, after making an uncomfortable decision at odds with his inner strivings, a person will tend subconsciously to refashion his beliefs to support the "reasonableness" of his decision.[102] At any rate, what we have dealt with in this chapter are some of the rationales, and rationalizations, which tend to entangle the prolongevitist in a net of fear, guilt and despair.

III. PROLONGEVITY LEGENDS

> And at the foot of that mount
> is a fair well. . . . Some men
> clepe it the well of youth . . .
> And men say, that that well
> cometh out of Paradise. . . .
>   Sir John Mandeville, *Travels*[1]

Myths and legends play an important role in the evolution of prolongevity thought. At the present time, the general public still does not distinguish always between legend and history, magic and science; in the

past such boundaries were less clearly demarcated and less regarded, and even scholars often were led astray. Before the development of modern archaeology, geology, history, and geography, it was difficult to deny the occurrence of miracles in the past or the existence of prodigies and marvels in remote areas of the earth, and traditions which we regard as mere legends served as bona fide inspiration for prolongevity concepts. If persons in other times or other places were reported to live a great deal longer than one's contemporaries, then one might hope to discover the vital secret and, thereby, be enabled to prolong life. When, in the course of history, the spurious nature of these traditions were recognized, they simply went underground and maintained their existence in the folklore of the uneducated, the fables of children, and the imaginative creations of artists and writers. From these sources, the ancient beliefs continue their influence, and it is a rare discussion on the subject of lengthening life which does not include at least a covert reference to Methuselah or the fountain of youth.

In an attempt to simplify a complex subject, this study will divide prolongevity legends into three main groups—the antediluvian, hyperborean, and fountain types.[2] The antediluvian theme is that people lived significantly longer in the past. The hyperborean tradition is that there are persons in other parts of the world who have unusually long lives. The fountain-type legend is based on the idea that it may be possible to prolong life by means of some remarkable substance. In addition to these three dominant types, several minor themes will be discussed briefly. Legends which include more than one theme will be classified according to which theme seems the more significant.

The word "prolongevity" is used rather loosely in this chapter in referring to legends in which longevity is extended by means other than ones directly under human control. An attempt has been made, however, to

---

[100] Jack Sheps, "Management of Fear of Death in Chronic Disease," *Jour. Amer. Geriatrics Society* **5** (1957): pp. 793–797.

[101] I. E. Alexander, R. S. Colley and A. M. Adlerstein, "Is Death a Matter of Indifference?" *Jour. Psychology* **43** (1957): 277–283. Two remarkable studies which add new dimensions to the psychology of death are Richard A. Kalish, "A Continuum of Subjectively Perceived Death," *The Gerontologist* **6** (1966): pp. 73–76, and Joseph C. Zinker and Stephen L. Fink, "The Possibility for Psychological Growth in a Dying Person," *Jour. General Psychology* **74** (1966): pp. 185–199.

[102] Leon Festinger, "Cognitive Dissonance," *Scientific American* **207**, 4 (1962): pp. 93–102.

[1] Sir John Mandeville, *Travels*, Library of English Classics (London, 1915), pp. 113–114.

[2] This classification is, I believe, original; I do not know of any previous study dealing in a comprehensive manner with prolongevity folklore. The most useful data came from articles in James Hastings, ed., *Encyclopedia of Religion and Ethics* (12 v., New York, 1908–1922); this work will be referred to collectively as "*E.R.E.*," while the articles will be cited separately. The other prime source was Eugene S. McCartney, "Longevity and Rejuvenation in Greek and Roman Folklore," *Papers Michigan Academy of Science, Arts and Letters* **5** (1925): pp. 37–72. A valuable work, too diffusely arranged, however, to be of much direct aid in this study, is Stith Thompson, *Motif-Index of Folk-Literature* (6 v., rev. ed., Bloomington, Indiana, 1955–1958); see, e.g., "immortality," "rejuvenation," "youth," etc. Fundamental for the comparative study of folklore but containing virtually nothing directly relative to the prolongation of life is James G. Frazer, *The Golden Bough: a Study in Magic and Religion* (12 v., London, 1900). Also useful for general orientation is Leo W. Simmons, *The Role of the Aged in Primitive Society* (New Haven, 1945) and Bessie Ellen Richardson, *Old Age Among the Ancient Greeks*, Johns Hopkins University Studies in Archaeology **16** (Baltimore, 1933).

keep the designation within bounds by bringing under consideration only those legends which reasonably might stimulate the idea of increasing longevity by human action.

THE ANTEDILUVIAN THEME [3]

The antediluvian theme, that people lived much longer in the past, is best exemplified by the familiar Hebrew tradition. In Genesis (5, 9:29) there are recorded the life spans of ten patriarchs who lived before the flood.

Adam	930	years
Seth	912	years
Enosh	905	years
Kenan	910	years
Mahalalel	895	years
Jared	962	years
Enoch	365	years
Methuselah	969	years
Lamech	777	years
Noah	950	years

The ages range from the 365 years of Enoch to the 969 years of Methuselah, whose name has become a byword for longevity.[4]

Legends of the antediluvian type frequently occur in the world's folklore. Among primitive peoples, for example, there appears the idea that mankind once possessed the means of avoiding death; for example, the Trobrianders, the Ainu and the Banks Islanders believed their forefathers had been able to rejuvenate themselves by shedding their skin like snakes.[5] Greek and Roman historical traditions refer to a number of persons of the past who attained prodigious longevity. In the material of this sort collected by Pliny, the ages range from one hundred fifty to eight hundred years.[6] In India, tradition describes primeval men of enormous longevity.[7]

These antediluvian traditions can be understood as a subsidiary variant of primitivism, the belief that, in general, things were much better at some time in the past.[8] Primitivist folklore usually includes a reference to long life spans. According to Hesiod, for example, the men

of the golden age never grew old, and when death came it was as gentle as sleep.[9]

Appearing in the holy Scriptures, the longevity records of the antediluvians posed a problem of interpretation for Jewish and Christian theologians. Three types of explanation were put forth—mythical, metaphorical, and literal.[10] The mythical interpretation denies them any historical validity. The metaphorical interpretation reasons that each patriarch symbolizes a tribe or dynasty or that the word "year" is used differently from our own. Neither of these explanations would generate ideas of prolongevity. Of more interest here is the literal interpretation exemplified by the Roman-Jewish historian, Josephus. In his work on Jewish antiquities, Josephus justified the longevity of the antediluvians on the grounds that they were "beloved of God" and had a diet conducive to long life, and he cited the traditions of Egypt, Babylonia, Phoenicia, and Greece to support his contention that "the ancients lived for a thousand years."[11] St. Augustine in The City of God argued at length in favor of a literal interpretation of the antediluvian data.[12]

From a literal interpretation of Old Testament chronology, support might be drawn for either apologism or meliorism. To some, the decrease in man's life span from above nine hundred to one hundred twenty years in Genesis (6:3) and to seventy or eighty years in Psalms (90:10) seemed an unmistakable indication that God's will was to shorten rather than lengthen earthly life. However, an unorthodox thinker like Roger Bacon was able to find inspiration in the long lives of the ancients. Bacon deduced that, if, after the Fall, men still were able to live almost a thousand years, then the short life span of his own times might be the result not of the will of God but of the ignorance of man.[13]

Although the age of gold usually was placed in the remote past, the idea was so attractive that it reappeared in other forms. It might be thought that in some far corner of the earth the age of gold continued its existence; this was the Abode-of-the-Blest theme which is discussed in the next section. Another belief was that the golden age was to return, perhaps in the near future. During the early years of the Roman Empire there was some hope that history, having run a full cycle, was about to be reborn.[14] The Hebrews, oppressed by for-

---

[3] The best orientation for the antediluvian theme, and also much of the legendary material itself, can be found in Arthur O. Lovejoy and George Boas, eds., *Primitivism and Related Ideas in Antiquity* (Baltimore, 1935), and George Boas, *Essays on Primitivism and Related Ideas in the Middle Ages* (Baltimore, 1948). See also, McCartney, *op. cit.* (see fn. 2), pp. 37–43.

[4] But note that six other patriarchs lived beyond nine hundred years.

[5] Simmons, *op. cit.* (see fn. 2), pp. 218–219.

[6] Pliny, *Natural History*, book 7, chap. 49 ("The Greatest Length of Life").

[7] Hermann Jacobi, "Ages of the World (Indian)," *E.R.E.* 1: pp. 200–202, and Louis de la Vallée Poussin, "Ages of the World (Buddhist)," *E.R.E.* 1: pp. 187–190.

[8] On primitivism, see Lovejoy and Boas, *op. cit.* and Boas, *op. cit.* (see fn. 3).

[9] See earlier, chap. II, section on myth and legend.

[10] C. van den Biesen, "Antediluvians," *Catholic Encyclopedia* (New York, 1907-1914) 1: pp. 551–553.

[11] Josephus, *Jewish Antiquities*, in *Josephus*, H. St. J. Thackeray and Ralph Marcus transl., Loeb Classical Library (9 v., London and New York, 1930) 4: pp. 51–53.

[12] Augustine, *The City of God*, book 15, sections 9–14.

[13] Tenney L. Davis, ed. and transl., *Roger Bacon's Letter Concerning the Marvelous Power of Art and of Nature and Concerning the Nullity of Magic* (Easton, Pa., London and Tokyo, 1923), pp. 35–37. For more on Bacon's rationale of prolongevitism, see later, chap. VI.

[14] Vergil, *Eclogues*, in *Virgil's Works*, J. W. Mackail, transl., Modern Library (New York, 1950), pp. 274–275.

eign rule, developed an urgent vision of a new golden age, which was to be ushered in by a Messiah, sent by God to establish an earthly paradise centered on Jerusalem. Then, among other marvels, the longevity of the patriarchs would be restored, so that a man of a hundred would be considered a mere child.[15]

> And they shall live a long life on earth,
> Such as thy fathers lived:
> And in their days shall no (sorrow) or plague
> Or torment or calamity touch them.[16]

Christianity transformed the role of the Messiah to one of suffering and redemption; nevertheless, the desire for an earthly paradise lived on in ideas of the Second Coming, which would inaugurate a thousand years (millennium) of earthly glory characterized by nearly all the traditional attributes of the golden-age theme.[17] Despite the disapproval of orthodox theologians, the history of Christianity has been marked by periodic recurrences of millennialist tendencies, most recently in the Social Gospel movement and in various Adventist sects.[18]

THE HYPERBOREAN THEME [19]

The Greek legend of the Hyperboreans is the prototype for the hyperborean theme, the idea that in some remote part of the world there are people who enjoy a remarkably long life. According to the traditions of ancient Greece, there dwells *hyper* (beyond) *Boreas* (the north wind) a fortunate people free from all natural ills.[20]

> . . . their hair crowned with golden bay-leaves they hold glad revelry; and neither sickness nor baneful eld mingleth among that chosen people; but, aloof from toil and conflict, they dwell afar. . . .[21]

Strabo stated that a longevity of a thousand years was attributed to the Hyperboreans, while Pliny wrote that they live to "an extreme old age" until, sated with life and luxury, they leap into the sea.[22]

So long as transport and communications remained difficult, it was easy for exaggerated ideas to arise concerning the longevity of persons in isolated localities. A life of one hundred fifty years could be ascribed to the inhabitants of Mount Tmolus in Asia Minor and four hundred years to those of Mount Athos in Greece. At the southern periphery of the world were the Ethiopians, living up to four hundred years; while in the farthest east were the Indian Cyrni, also living four hundred years, and the people of Ceylon, whose life was "prolonged to an extreme length." [23]

The hyperborean legend, however, transcends the speculations of travelers and geographers and is best understood as a variation of one of the basic themes of world folklore—the Abode of the Blest.[24] Many cultures have a tradition that somewhere on this earth there is a veritable paradise. The idea seems to have arisen in part from the widespread belief that somewhere the age of gold still might be in existence. The abode of the blest must be distinguished carefully from places where people go after death or places in other worlds; the persons in the abode of the blest may have supernatural characteristics, but they are alive and dwell somewhere in this world. The abode-of-the-blest concept is a comparatively naive notion hovering on the borderline between the natural and the supernatural. With the further evolution of religion, the earthly paradise develops into a reward of righteous souls after death and finally is removed altogether from earth and placed in the heavens.

In Greek folklore there are two different abodes of the blest: the land of the Hyperboreans and the Isles of the Blest.[25] The story of the Hyperboreans seems to have originated in connection with the early migration of Greek tribes from the North.[26] The Isles of the Blest have a more supernatural quality and are inhabited by the semi-divine race which fought at Thebes and Troy.[27] These islands, "untouched by sorrow," usually were located in the Atlantic Ocean.

The traditions of ancient India speak of the Uttarakurus, a fortunate race living in the far north and enjoying a marvelous longevity; the similarity of this legend with the Greek Hyperboreans already was recognized in ancient times.[28] In the land of the Uttarakurus

[15] Isaiah 65: 20.
[16] Enoch 25: 6, in *Apocrypha and Pseudepigrapha of the Old Testament*, Robert H. Charles, ed. (2 v., Oxford, 1913) 2: p. 205.
[17] J. F. Bethune-Baker, *Introduction to the Early History of Christian Doctrine* (5th ed., London, 1933), pp. 68-71.
[18] An example of Christian millennialism blending with the idea of progress and the idea of prolongevity is Joseph Priestley; see later, chap. VIII, introduction.
[19] The best guide to hyperborean-type legends is the section "Blest, Abode of the," *E.R.E.* 2: pp. 680-710; hereafter referred to as "Blest." There is a survey of this sort of theme in Kuno Meyer and Alfred Nutt, *The Voyage of Bran, Son of Febal, to the Land of the Living*, Grimm Library 4 (London, 1895), pp. 105-331. A good bit of material also can be found in Lovejoy and Boas, *op. cit.*, and Boas, *op. cit.* (see fn. 3).
[20] Edward Washburn Hopkins, "Hyperboreans," *E.R.E.* 7: pp. 58-59, and Lovejoy and Boas, *op. cit.* (see fn. 3), pp. 304-314.
[21] Pindar, *Pythian Odes*, 10, in *The Odes of Pindar*, Sir John Sandys, transl., Loeb Classical Library (London and New York, 1919), p. 293.
[22] Strabo, *Geography*, book 15, chap. 1, section 57 and Pliny, *op. cit.* (see fn. 6), book 4, chap. 26 ("Scythia"). *Cf.* the

"fullness-of-life" concept of the Stoics and Epicureans; see earlier, chap. II.
[23] Pliny, *op. cit.* (see fn. 6), book 7, chap. 2 ("The Wonderful Forms of Different Nations") and chap. 49 ("The Greatest Length of Life").
[24] See earlier, fn. 19.
[25] Frederick W. Hall, "Blest (Greek and Roman)," *E.R.E.* 2: pp. 696-698.
[26] Hopkins, *op. cit.* (see fn. 20).
[27] See earlier, chap. II, section on myth and legend.
[28] Hermann Jacobi, "Blest (Hindu)," *E.R.E.* 2: pp. 698-700 and Louis de la Vallée Poussin, "Blest (Buddhist)," *E.R.E.* 2: pp. 687-689. The Uttarakurus were referred to by the Greeks as "Attacori"; Pliny, *op. cit.* (see fn. 6), book 4, chap. 26 ("Scythia"), and book 6, chap. 20 ("The Seres").

grows the magic "Jambu" tree, whose fruit has the property of conferring immunity from illness and old age, and, by means of this fruit, they lengthen their lives to a thousand years or even, in some accounts, to eleven thousand years. Their sensuous pleasures make the visions of modern utopians seem pallid; among other things, their realm includes landscapes of precious stones and trees from whose branches grow beautiful maidens! As is usual in abode-of-the-blest legends, the status of the Uttarakurus remains ambiguous, for in some respects they seem identified with certain rather ordinary tribes of the Himalayas, but, at the other extreme, they become supernatural beings whose land is absolutely inaccessible to mortal men.

Greatly prolonged life also is a feature of Persian, Teutonic, Japanese, Hebrew, and Chinese versions of the abode of the blest.[29] A span of three hundred years is granted to the inhabitants of the "Land of Yima," which ancient Persian lore locates somewhere in the North, perhaps underground. Also in the North and probably underground is the Teutonic "Land of Living Men," but here there is no age or death at all, and the residents are a race of giants who welcome daring mortals. A Japanese version is the island of Horaisan occasionally reached by mortals, who find a land of eternal spring untouched by sickness, age, or death. Hebrew folklore also includes a remnant of the golden age, the Garden of Eden, where man dwelt on intimate terms with God and enjoyed a deathless life in a land of beauty and abundance. After the Fall, the tree of life is guarded by an angel with flaming sword, but the earthly paradise, located in the East near the Tigris and Euphrates rivers, continues to play a role in legends, especially, as will be seen, in those dealing with the fountain of youth. The hyperborean theme in China will be described in the chapter on Taoist theories about prolongevity.

The most vivid hyperborean-type legends were those of the Celts of Western Europe, describing an earthly paradise known as *Tir na nOg* (the Land of Youth) and various other names.[30] A number of stories, the best known of which is the "Voyage of Bran," recount the adventures of mortals seeking an island or series of islands in the West where the golden age still exists. Those who dwell there are supernatural beings, but a few favored mortals are allowed to enter. The chief attraction of the "Land of Youth" is the immunity from aging and death, obtained by eating certain enchanted foods or by using a magic cauldron. The country is rich in other delights: the handsome appearance of the inhabitants, the splendid landscape resonant with music, the lovemaking, and the plentiful supply of luxuries.

After the conversion of the Celts to Christianity, these pagan dreamlands retained their influence in such stories as the voyage of St. Brendan, one of the most popular of medieval sagas. And the Christian heaven assumed a more sensuous and materialistic aspect among the Celts than among other peoples.

Legends of the hyperborean and abode-of-the-blest type long served as a stimulus to geographical exploration. Despite the scepticism of such scholars as Strabo and Pliny, the Ancient World remained rather credulous as to the identification of various real Atlantic islands with the fabled earthly paradise.[31] During the Middle Ages, the attractions of such legendary places as the Isles of the Blest, St. Brendan's Island, Avalon, Atlantis, and Antilia became blended and spread an aura of glamor over Atlantic voyages.[32] Columbus, in 1498, on his third voyage, concluded that he had located the Terrestrial Paradise along the coast of Venezuela near the island of Trinidad. The four great rivers which empty into the Gulf of Paria he identified as the traditional rivers of Paradise: the Tigris, Euphrates, Nile, and Ganges. And in the distance were three mountains, at the summit of which must be Paradise itself.[33]

As the earth became almost completely mapped out and explored, the influence of hyperborean legends continued in a more indirect way. The Hyperboreans and the Uttarakurus had provided subjects for at least two ancient Greek writers of utopian romances, Amometus and Hecataeus (of Abdera), and the prolongation of life was to be a feature of utopian thought up to our own day.[34] An example of the hyperborean topic in contemporary fiction is the novel (and motion picture) *Lost Horizon* dealing with "Shangri La," a peaceful refuge in the Himalayas, where the life span is much longer than in the outside world.[35] The persistence of hyperboreanism in the popular mind again was revealed, when, in 1956, the visit to the United States by a Colombian Indian, alleged to be 167 years old, aroused public interest.[36] The last refuge for the hyperboreans

---

[29] Louis H. Gray, "Blest (Persian)," *E.R.E.* **2**: pp. 702–704; John A. MacCulloch, "Blest (Teutonic)," *E.R.E.* **2**: pp. 707–710, and "Blest (Japanese)," *E.R.E.* **2**: pp. 700–702; George A. Barton, "Blest (Semitic)," *E.R.E.* **2**: pp. 704–706.

[30] John A. MacCulloch, "Blest (Celtic)," *E.R.E.* **2**: pp. 689–696, and Meyer and Nutt, *op. cit.* (see fn. 19), pp. 1–104.

[31] Strabo, *Geography*, book 1, chap. 1, sections 4 and 5; book 3, chap. 2, section 13 and Pliny, *op. cit.* (see fn. 6), book 6, chap. 37 ("The Fortunate Islands"). *Cf.* Plutarch, "Sertorius," in *Plutarch's Lives*, Bernadotte Perrin, transl., Loeb Classical Library (11 v., London and New York, 1919) **8**: pp. 21–23.

[32] See "Antilia," "Atlantis," "Avalon," "Brendan," *Encyclopedia Britannica* (11th ed., 1910).

[33] Samuel Eliot Morison, *Admiral of the Ocean Sea: a Life of Christopher Columbus* (Boston, 1942), pp. 556–558; and Peter Martyr d'Anghiera, *De orbe novo*, Francis A. MacNutt, transl. (2 v., New York, 1912) **1**: p. 139.

[34] Hall, *op. cit.* (see fn. 25). For English translation of the remaining fragments of Hecataeus of Abdera's "Hyperboreans," see Lovejoy and Boas, *op. cit.* (see fn. 3), pp. 307–310. The prolongevitism of the modern utopians will be analyzed in my work, *Death and Progress: the Rise of Secular Salvation*.

[35] James Hilton, *Lost Horizon* (New York, 1933); movie directed by Frank Capra, 1938.

[36] *New York Times*, 9-28-56: p. 29. See also the report on long life in Hunza, a Himalayan principality; 7-11-60, p. 10.

would seem to be outer space. The American Darwinist C. A. Stephens speculated about a possible immortal race on some other planet and made this the subject of a science-fiction story.[37]

THE FOUNTAIN THEME

The third main type of prolongevity legend is based on the idea that there exists some unusual substance which has the property of greatly increasing the length of life. The prototype of this theme is the legend of a fountain whose waters bring about rejuvenation, the restoration of youth. The legend has been made familiar to generations of American schoolchildren in the story of Juan Ponce de León, whose quest for the fountain led accidentally to the discovery of Florida in 1513.[38]

The earliest account of Ponce de León's adventure was published in 1535 in the *General History of the Indies* by Oviedo, who had served as a Spanish official in the New World. He wrote that Ponce de León was

. . . seeking that fountain of Biminie that the Indians had given it to be understood would renovate or resprout and refresh the age and forces of he [*sic*] who drank or bathed himself in that fountain.[39]

Gomara, whose *History of the Indies* was published in 1552–1553, depicted Ponce de León as

. . . fitting out two caravels to seek the island of Boica where, according to the Indians, there was the fountain which transformed the aged to youths.[40]

A somewhat different version of the expedition was given in 1575 in the *Memoir* of Fontaneda, a Spaniard who was held captive for twenty-seven years by Florida Indians. Fontaneda connected Ponce de León with the tradition that the much-venerated Jordan River (flowing out of Eden) might be found in the Indies.

Juan Ponz [*sic*] de León . . . went to Florida in search of the River Jordan . . . that he might become young from bathing in such a stream.[41]

Besides illustrating the legend of the fountain of youth, the story of Ponce de León itself represents something of a legend. Over the years, imaginative writers transformed the tough, fifty-five-year-old adventurer into a sentimental old man whose decrepit condition prevented

him from satisfying his beautiful young wife.[42] A nineteenth-century painting depicts a senile Ponce de León with flowing white beard dreaming of youthful houris cavorting in a forest spring.[43] In reaction to these sensational accounts, some scholars have gone to the other extreme and dismissed the whole thing as "discredited" and "ridiculous." [44]

Although we cannot be certain to what degree, if any, Ponce de León's expedition was stimulated by the desire to find a fountain of youth, there is no reason to exclude such a motivation. Interest in the fountain of youth had reached an apex in the fourteenth and fifteenth centuries, and the discovery of America gave a new impetus to the tradition in the early years of the sixteenth century. Peter Martyr d'Anghiera, a member of the Council of the Indies and in close contact with Spanish explorers and officials, testifies to the impact of the legend. When the first fountain-of-youth reports came in from the colonies about 1514, Peter Martyr wrote a letter to the Pope saying,

Let not Your Holiness believe this to be a hasty or foolish opinion, for the story has been most seriously told to all the court, and made such an impression that the entire populace, and even people superior by birth and influence, accepted it as a proven fact.[45]

At first, the pious scholar avowed his own opinion to be that the power of rejuvenation is not to be found in nature but is reserved to God. Later, his caution decreased when three high officials returned from the Indies with a firm belief in the existence of the fountain. One of them had a servant whose father allegedly had been revivified by the marvelous spring. Peter Martyr now reasoned that if, according to natural philosophers, Mother Nature provides means of rejuvenation to dumb animals like the snake, the eagle, and the crow, why should she not also create similar bounties for man?[46]

The fountain-of-youth legend of Ponce de León's and Peter Martyr's times has been traced by scholars to two ancient origins, the Hindu Pool of Youth and the Hebrew River of Immortality.[47] The Hindu contribution is embodied in the legend of Cyavana, which is at least as old as 700 B.C. and probably considerably older. According to the story, Cyavana, the aged and venerable priest of a Hindu king, comes into conflict with the

---

[37] C. A. Stephens, *Natural Salvation, the Message of Science* (Norway Lake, Maine, 1903), pp. 77, 121 and "The Platinum Spheroid," *Long Life* 2 (1896) : pp. 139–186. For similar ideas from the other end of the religious spectrum, the Jesuit; see *New York Times*, 8-7-60: p. 14.

[38] On the Spanish conquistadors and the fountain of youth, see Eug. Beauvois, "La Fontaine de jouvence et le Jourdain dans les traditions des Antilles et de la Floride," *Le Muséon* (Louvain) 3 (1884) : pp. 404–429.

[39] *Ibid.*, pp. 416–417, and Edward W. Lawson, *The Discovery of Florida and its Discoverer Juan Ponce de León* (St. Augustine, 1946), p. 108 .

[40] Beauvois, *op. cit.* (see fn. 38), p. 415.

[41] Hernando d'Escalente Fontaneda, *Memoir*, Buckingham Smith, transl. (Miami, 1944), pp. 14–15.

[42] E.g., *ibid.*, passage quoted by the editors, p. 46.

[43] Carita Doggett Corse, *The Fountain of Youth* (St. Augustine, 1937), p. 6. Once again we note the persistent relationship of prolongevity and sex.

[44] *Columbia Encyclopedia*, William Bridgewater and Elizabeth J. Sherwood, eds. (New York, 1950), p. 1576 and Fontaneda, *op. cit.* (see fn. 41), comment by the editors on p. 47.

[45] Peter Martyr d'Anghiera, *op. cit.* (see fn. 33), 1 : p. 274.

[46] *Ibid.* 2 : pp. 293–295. *Cf.*, later, the "phoenix theme."

[47] On the fountain of youth, see Edward Washburn Hopkins, "Fountain of Youth," *E.R.E.* 6: pp. 115–116, and "The Fountain of Youth," *Jour. Amer. Oriental Society* 26 (1905) : pp. 1–67. See also, Louis Masson, "La Fontaine de jouvence," *Aesculape* (Paris) 27 (1937) : pp. 244–251, and 28 (1938) : pp. 16–23.

king's haughty sons. To pacify the offended sage, the king gives his own daughter Sukanya to be the wife of Cyavana. At this point there appear the two Asvins, demi-gods who go about the earth practicing medicine. They are much taken with the attractive young Sukanya, and, casting scorn on her decrepit husband, they try to seduce her; but the dutiful girl chooses to remain faithful to her senile husband. Cyavana decides to capitalize on the situation by offering to reveal certain religious secrets to the Asvins in exchange for rejuvenation. The bargain is sealed, and the Asvins take Cyavana to the Pool of Youth.

Thereupon Cyavana quickly entered the water in his desire for beauty. The Asvins also then went into the stream. A moment after, they came up out of the stream, divinely fair, all of them, and youthful, (wearing) brilliant earrings.[48]

This Hindu fable probably was transmitted to medieval Europe by either the Arabs or the Nestorian Christians of the Near East.

Blending easily with this Hindu motif of rejuvenation was the ancient Hebrew legend of a River of Immortality which conferred eternal life, although not necessarily renewed youth. Genesis (2:10) mentions a river flowing out of Eden, and Psalms (36:9) refers rather figuratively to a "fountain of life." From these slender remarks, together with the "river of the water of life" in Revelation (22:1), there evolved an elaborate branch of Christian symbolism, in which Christ was identified with the Fountain of Life.[49] At the same time, these Biblical words inspired a legend that there existed a real fountain flowing out of the Terrestrial Paradise to come within the reach of mortal men. Examples of that idea will be seen in the medieval Alexander romances. Even within Christianity the Fountain of Life sometimes possessed physical as well as spiritual attributes, especially in the Byzantine Church where the cult was associated with actual springs having miraculous healing powers.[50] Indicative of this ambiguity is the story, told at the Byzantine fountain shrine of Balukli, relating the revival of a dead fish, a theme which recurs in secular stories about the fountain of youth.

In ancient Greek and Roman writings there are two interesting references to fountains with prolongevity properties. Pausanias, in his travel guidebook to Greece, noted that near the seaport of Nauplia there was a spring in which, according to local religious belief, Hera, the wife of Zeus, bathed every year in order to renew her maidenhood.[51] In later times, the spring became identified with a heavily ornamented fountain

in the garden of a nunnery, which had a shrine dedicated to the Byzantine cult of the Water of Life.[52]

The other classical reference, less supernatural in tone, is in Herodotus' account of some agents sent by the Persian emperor to spy out the land of Ethiopia.[53] The spies showed disbelief when the Ethiopian king claimed for his people a life expectancy of one hundred twenty years. To overcome their doubts, the king led them to a spring with waters of a strangely oily and fragrant quality.

So frail, the spies said, was the water, that nothing would float on it, neither wood nor anything lighter than wood, but all sank to the bottom. If this water be truly such as they say, it is likely that their constant use of it makes the people long-lived.[54]

This passage recalls the cold-dry theory of aging discussed in the previous chapter, according to which senility was caused by the loss of "vital" moisture. The implication of Herodotus' statement is that, if the waters of the Ethiopian spring are oilier and lighter than ordinary moisture, then they partake of the characteristics of "vital" moisture and, by frequent contact with the body, might actually lengthen life.

Despite these intriguing remarks by Herodotus and Pausanias, the idea of a fountain of youth remained alien to Greco-Roman culture, and the only Classical contribution to the legend was an indirect one—the story of Glaukus. In an elegant version of the fable, Glaukus, a fisherman, came upon a hitherto-unexplored meadow on the shore of the sea.[55] Having spread his catch of fish on the ground, he was amazed to see them nibble at the grass, become wonderfully revivified, and leap into the water. Following their example, Glaukus ate of the herbs and plunged into the waters where he became an immortal sea-divinity. As part of the transition, his beard and body turned to a greenish color, a phenomenon which explains his name, glaukos or "bluish green."

The Glaukus legend was utilized in the tales of Alexander the Great's search for the fountain of youth, a colorful adventure concocted by imaginative writers in the ancient Near East.[56] In one version, Alexander has a cook who, while cleaning a dried fish in a spring, is astounded to see it leap into life. Realizing that this must be the Fountain of Life, the cook bathes in the waters and becomes immortal. Alexander, unable to dis-

---

[48] Hopkins, op. cit. (see fn. 47), p. 52.

[49] Evelyn Underhill, "The Fountain of Life: an Iconographical Study," Burlington Magazine 17 (1910): pp. 99–109.

[50] Charles Talbot, "The Fountain of Life: a Greek Version," Bull. History Medicine 31 (1957): pp. 1–16.

[51] Pausanias, Description of Greece, W. H. S. Jones, transl., Loeb Classical Library (5 v., London and New York, 1918) 1: p. 455 ("Corinth," section 38).

[52] Talbot, op. cit. (see fn. 50), pp. 15–16.

[53] A. D. Godley, transl., Herodotus, Loeb Classical Library (4 v., London and New York, 1921) 2: pp. 27–33 (book 3, sections 20–24).

[54] Ibid., p. 31.

[55] Ovid, Metamorphoses, Frank Justus Miller, transl., Loeb Classical Library (2 v., London and New York, 1916) 2: pp. 293–297 (last part of book 13).

[56] The best available introduction to the Alexander legends is Armand Abel, Le Roman d'Alexandre, Collections Lebeque et nationale 112 (Brussels, 1955); on the Near Eastern origins of the tale, see pp. 11, 14–15, 24–27.

cover the fountain himself, decides to kill the cook, but, finding him invulnerable to death, has him thrown into the sea where he lives on as a demon. The fountain in this story is located near Paradise.

In Arabic legend, Alexander's cook was replaced by el Khidr, "the Green One," obviously modeled on Glaukus.[57] El Khidr was the most popular figure in Islamic folklore, playing a role similar to that of Elijah in Jewish traditions as a mortal whose saintliness was rewarded by direct accession to immortal life without the intervention of death. In Arabic stories el Khidr appears as a general and trusted adviser of Alexander; in fact, the Muslim el Khidr tends to assume greater importance than the pagan Alexander. In one version an angel tells Alexander of the existence of the "Well of the Water of Life" in Arabia.[58] The well is discovered accidentally by el Khidr when he washes a dried fish in the water and sees it brought back to life. El Khidr bathes in the water, becomes immortal, and, in the process, his body and garments turn bluish green. Already in the Koran, there is a rather enigmatic passage which refers to el Khidr's discovery of the Water of Life.[59]

The Alexander legend attained its finest literary expression in the Romance of Alexander, a long epic-like poem composed in twelfth-century France by Lambert le Tors and Alexandre de Bernay.[60] In one of the episodes, Alexander, on an expedition near India, encounters four aged men who tell him of three different miraculous fountains.[61] The first, which restores the dead to life, is discovered when two boiled fish accidentally are dropped into it and are resuscitated.[62] The second fountain, which confers immortality, is only accessible once each year. As luck would have it, an ordinary soldier comes upon the fountain and bathes in it, thereby blocking the chances of Alexander. For punishment, the crafty fellow is sealed up inside a stone column. Finally the expedition reaches the third fountain, which has powers of rejuvenation. All, including the four senile guides, bathe in this genuine fountain of youth and are returned to the condition of men of thirty

years of age.[63] This last fountain is described as originating from the Euphrates, one of the four rivers of Paradise. A similar fountain appears in another popular medieval romance, Huon de Bordeaux.[64]

By the time of Ponce de León, the fountain-of-youth idea must have become familiar to everyone in Western Europe. In addition to the romances, the motif often occurred in medieval folk tales, especially in variations of the three-brothers story, in which an aged king sends his sons on a quest for some magic, rejuvenating water in a distant land.[65] The fountain also was frequently a theme of artists, the most famous version being the lively painting by Lucas Cranach in 1546.[66] Finally, there was the medieval travel literature, identified with the names of Prester John and Sir John Mandeville, which described a fountain of youth issuing from Paradise and accessible in "India."[67] It is clear that the Spanish explorers of Ponce de León's day might very well have had the fountain of youth in mind as they sailed to "the Indies."

Marvelous waters, however, represent only one variety of the fountain-type legend, which was defined as being based on the idea that there exists a substance with the property of significantly prolonging life. Besides the water of the fountain of youth there are a host of other prolongevity substances which appear in legends. It will not be possible to describe and analyze all these materials in detail. Instead, three groupings will be suggested by which these substances can be organized and explained.

The first grouping would be substances with divine properties. Included here would be the life-prolonging food and drink of the gods, for example, the Greek ambrosia and nectar, the soma of the Hindus and Persians, and the octli of ancient Mexico and Peru.[68] Such materials exist in a hazy borderland between the natural and supernatural, at times being ethereal and unobtainable, and then again being identified with such mundane substances as honey or the fermented juice of the soma plant. Closely related to these foods of the gods are the foods of the blest in the various terrestrial

[57] On el Khidr, see the excellent account by I. Friedlaender, "Khidr," E.R.E. 7: pp. 693–695. This is the source for the above story of Alexander's cook.

[58] E. A. Wallis Budge, The Life and Exploits of Alexander the Great, Being a Series of Translations of the Ethiopic Histories of Alexander (London, 1896), pp. 261–271.

[59] Sura 18 ("The Cave"): 61–95. In these lines, Alexander is represented by "Moses" and by "Dhu'l-Qarneyn" (the two-horned one), while el Khidr is "one of Our slaves." Cf. Friedlaender, op. cit. (see fn. 57), p. 694, and Abel, op. cit. (see fn. 56), p. 119, n. 9.

[60] Lewis Spence, A Dictionary of Medieval Romance and Romance Writers (London and New York, 1913), pp. 5–6, 218–219, 318–319.

[61] Paul Meyer, Alexandre le Grand dans la littérature française du moyen âge, Bibliothèque française du moyen âge 2 (Paris, 1886): pp. 174 ff.

[62] For more about resuscitation, see later, chap. VIII.

[63] Cf. earlier, chap. II, for Avicenna's choice of thirty as the high point of human physical development.

[64] Meyer, op. cit. (see fn. 61), pp. 184–185.

[65] Hopkins, op. cit. (see fn. 47), 12 ff. See also "The Water of Life" in Joseph Scharl, ed., Grimm's Fairy Tales (London, 1948), pp. 449–455.

[66] Reproduced in most books on Cranach. Good copies also may be seen in Frederic D. Zeman, "Studies in the Medical History of Old Age: the Medieval Period," Jour. M:. Sinai Hosp. (N. Y.) 12 (1945): p. 789, and Sona Rosa Burstein, "The Quest for Rejuvenation," Geriatrics 10 (1955): p. 537. There is a great deal on the fountain in art in Masson, op. cit. (see fn. 47).

[67] Hopkins, op. cit (see fn. 47), pp. 21–22.

[68] McCartney, op. cit. (see fn. 2), pp. 45–46, and Edward Washburn Hopkins, "Soma," E.R.E. 11: pp. 685–687. There seems to be a continuity in religious interpretation of the "miracle" of fermentation from its discovery in neolithic times down to the present-day communion with bread and wine.

paradises, for example, the fruit of the "Jambu" tree of the Uttarakurus, or the fruit of the tree of life in the garden of Eden. To the extent that it derives from the River of Immortality, flowing out of Eden, the water of the fountain of youth may be classsified in this category. One of the most interesting of these objects is the Celtic "magic cauldron" which conferred both abundance of food and bodily immortality. At first the reward of pagan adventurers reaching the abode of the blest, the "magic cauldron" later evolved into the Holy Grail sought by medieval Christian knights.[69]

Secondly, there are the prolongevity substances with empirical qualities. It is alleged that they simply have been found to work, and no further explanation is required. For example, by the "cut-and-try" method of ordinary human experience, a great many plant materials have been found to have beneficial medical properties. Starting from that basis, one might imagine an herb with the power of prolonging life, perhaps indefinitely, as the grassy herb of the Glaukus legend. Similarly, there have been known from the earliest times thermal and mineral springs with genuine healing effects for various diseases. Carrying this fact a few steps further, one might speculate about the existence of a spring with the attribute of combatting old age, as, for example, the "Pool of Youth" of Hindu folklore.

Comprising the third group would be the substances which prolong life because of their magical qualities. According to the implicit principles of magic, humans can produce great effects upon nature by elementary processes of contact and imitation.[70] If, for example, certain animals were considered to be long-lived, it follows from the laws of magic that contact with those animals will lengthen life. Thus, when Medea, of Greek legend, prepared a rejuvenating brew, she utilized such items as the skin of a snake, the liver of a stag, and the head of a crow.[71] Similarly, if water renews the crops in the great river valleys of the Near East, then, by the rules of magic, water also may reinvigorate the body, as in the fountain of youth. Along lines such as these, explanations can be found for the life-prolonging powers of fire, precious gems, and a myriad of prolongevity substances, charms, and ceremonies which appear in the world's folklore.[72]

MISCELLANEOUS THEMES

Outside the definition of prolongevity, as extension of life by human action, are the legends in which immortality or rejuvenation are conferred directly by divine fiat. Of interest, however, is the story of Hercules, the semi-divine hero, whose exploits finally earned him a place among the deathless gods.[73] Some of the feats of Hercules, the most popular figure of Greek folklore, illustrate tendencies among the Greeks favoring meliorism and the prolongation of life. It was Hercules who freed Prometheus, symbol of human activism and pride, and it was Hercules who wrestled with Death and forced him to restore to life the wife of Admetus. Another conquest by Hercules, portrayed in a number of works of art, was his victorious battle with Geras, the ugly personification of old age.[74] Suitably enough, when he took his place among the immortal gods, Hercules was married to Hebe, the goddess of youth.

More directly tied to prolongevity are legends characterized by what may be called the phoenix theme, the idea that there exist animals enjoying a much greater length of life than man.[75] According to Hesiod, for example, the crow lives nine times as long as man, the stag thirty-six times as long, the raven 108, and the "phoenix," a miraculous bird of Egyptian folklore, 1,080. The remarkable longevity of some animals was explained by their possessing methods of rejuvenation. The snake was thought to renew its youth by shedding its skin, while the aged eagle restored its vigor by flying to India where it plunged into the fountain of youth.[76] The phoenix theme provided a challenging stimulus to prolongevity efforts, since it seemed humiliating that man should be outlived by any of the brute animals.

Recent developments in physiology call to mind another legendary motif which may be named the Endymion theme, the belief that youth might be preserved by one's falling into a trance-like sleep. In Greek tradition, the Moon fell in love with Endymion, a youth of surpassing beauty.[77] As a reward, or in other accounts out of jealousy, Zeus placed him in a condition of eternal slumber in which he remains forever young and handsome. A variant of the Endymion theme is the story of "Sleeping Beauty," familiar to modern readers in the version of Grimm, in which the princess and her court are doomed to sleep a hundred years until rescued by a venturesome prince.[78] Such tales reflect human observation of animal hibernation and blend with age-old speculation about the possibility of suspended animation,

[69] MacCulloch, op. cit. (see fn. 30), p. 694.

[70] Frazer, op. cit. (see fn. 2) 1: pp. 52 ff.

[71] McCartney, op. cit. (see fn. 2), p. 55.

[72] E.g., Hopkins, op. cit. (see fn. 47), pp. 3-4, n. 4. Also, see later, Taoist dietary techniques (chap. V) and Taoist and Latin alchemy (chap. VI).

[73] Edith Hamilton, Mythology (New York, 1953), pp. 167-172.

[74] Richardson, op. cit. (see fn. 2), pp. 73-76.

[75] McCartney, op. cit. (see fn. 2), pp. 42-45. For Chinese versions of the phoenix theme, see later, chap. IV, section on magic and folklore. For contemporary views, see Alex Comfort, "The Life Span of Animals," Scientific American 205, 2 (1961): pp. 108-119. On how belief in the existence of the phoenix stimulated early-modern Western exploration of the East Indies, see Thomas P. Harrison, "Bird of Paradise: Phoenix Redivivus," Isis 51 (1960): pp. 173-180.

[76] On the eagle, see Hopkins, op. cit. (see fn. 47), pp. 38-42. Dante used the eagle symbol in The Divine Comedy, canto 9 of "Purgatorio," the Carlyle-Wicksteed transl., Modern Library (New York, 1950), pp. 243 and 246 n. 3.

[77] McCartney, op. cit. (see fn. 2), pp. 46-47.

[78] E.g., "Little Briar-Rose" in Scharl, op. cit. (see fn. 65), pp. 237-241.

a phenomenon which now seems on the threshold of scientific possibility.[79] Since the rediscovery in 1948 of the protective effects of glycerol (first reported by Jean Rostand in 1946), a series of notable experiments has demonstrated that rats and hamsters can be kept frozen for an hour or two and then restored to life unharmed.[80] Since the frozen body does not age, this work opens up the possibility that some day human beings may be kept in biostasis (suspended animation) for long periods of time. Myth and legend have played a useful role in preparing the public for this development; as an eminent scientist has remarked,

the idea of biostasis of the whole body, macabre at first sight, holds nothing new in principle, being woven into the fabric of countless human beliefs, from the resurrection of the dead to the awakening of the Sleeping Beauty.[81]

CONCLUSION

In the previous chapter it was shown that the apologist outlook early achieved dominance in philosophy, religion, and science, that is, in educated and intellectual circles, which in ancient and medieval times comprised only a small part of the population. In this chapter we have seen that, despite the rationalizing of the apologists, there existed a great profusion of legendary material expressing the basic human wish for prolonged life on this earth. In folklore, with its free expression of wishes, the basic aspirations and dreams of the unlettered populace were able to come to the fore. These primitive forms of the idea of prolongevity were fascinating even to scholars and clerics who were committed to the tenets of apologism. It is as though apologism controlled the Super-ego, while meliorism and prolongevity subsisted in the half-conscious twilight of the Id.

In addition to expressing and keeping alive a deep human yearning, prolongevity legends served as a stimulus and, at times, as a guide to prolongevity research. In the course of this chapter, a number of illustrations of this influence have been mentioned, for example, the occurrence of the antediluvian theme in Roger Bacon's work and the appearance of the hyperborean theme in the work of C. A. Stephens. In subsequent chapters, other examples will be pointed out in which prolongevity legends inspired or pervaded efforts to prolong life.

The most significant types of prolongevity lore in that regard are the empirical and magic varieties of the fountain-type legend. From the empirical search for herbs and drugs, and from the magical quest for potent analogies in nature, there arose pharmacy and alchemy, and from those early studies there developed ultimately the modern sciences of pharmacology and biochemistry with their promise of truly effective weapons in the effort to overcome senescence.

IV. TAOIST PROLONGEVITISM IN THEORY

The *hsien* books say: Who eats the elixir of life and guards the One (Tao), lives as long as heaven exists, he revives the constituents of his nature, stores up his breath, and thus lengthens his life indefinitely.

Ko Hung, fourth century [1]

One of the most thought-provoking features of the evolution of prolongevitism is the striking contrast between China and the West. In ancient and early-medieval China, a great philosophico-religious system, Taoism, was allied with prolongevitism. In the West there was no development of comparable magnitude; [2] indeed, as was demonstrated in chapter II, the leading intellectual currents were extensively infiltrated with apologism, the belief that prolongevity is neither possible nor desirable.

That is not to say that prolongevitist tendencies were totally lacking in ancient Western civilization. As was seen in chapter III, magical and religious forms of prolongevitism played a significant role in Western folklore. Religious prolongevitism also appeared in the ideas of the ancient Hebrews (*cf.,* chap. II). And one can cite examples of natural prolongevitism: the Smith Papyrus of ancient Egypt included a recipe "for transforming an old man into a youth," [3] and the Greek philosopher Empedokles promised his disciples a knowledge of drugs to combat aging.[4]

But in the West these tendencies remained fragmentary, while in China they were richly elaborated and made the subject of entire treatises. In the West, prolongevity was pushed to the periphery of the intellectual world or even driven underground, while in China it occupied a central position and attracted the attention of famous scholars, influential statesmen and, at times, the emperors themselves. Taoism, for the first time in

---

[79] On speculation about suspended animation and "anabiosis," see later, chap. VIII, section on Franklin.

[80] A. S. Parkes, "Preservation of Tissue *in Vitro* for the study of Ageing," *Ciba Foundation Colloquia on Aging* 1: *General Aspects* (Boston, 1955), pp. 162–169.

[81] *Ibid.*, p. 169. See also, Robert C. W. Ettinger, *The Prospect of Immortality* (New York, 1964), for a forceful account of low-temperature biostasis; there are prefaces by Jean Rostand and Gerald J. Gruman. In addition, Ettinger has written, "The Frozen Christian," *Christian Century* 82 (1965): pp. 1313–1315, and "Science and Immortality," *Yale Scientific Magazine* 40, 7 (1966): pp. 5–8; 20. A fascinating store of material can be found in *Life Extension Society Newsletter* (Washington) 1 ff. (1964 ff.); title changed to *Freeze-Wait-Reanimate* as of 2 (1965).

[1] Ko Hung, *Pao-p'u Tzu*, chap. 3, Eugene Feifel, transl., *Monumenta Serica* (Peking) 6 (1941): p. 183.

[2] *Cf.* Joseph Needham, *Science and Civilization in China* (Cambridge, 1954 ff.) 2: p. 139, especially "note d"; this work hereafter will be referred to as "Needham, *SCC.*" There is a sensitive and sophisticated study of the humanistic, this-worldly basis of Chinese prolongevitism by Ying-shih Yü, "Life and Immortality in the Mind of Han China," *Harvard Jour. Asiatic Studies* 25 (1964–1965): pp. 80–122.

[3] James H. Breasted, *The Edwin Smith Surgical Papyrus* (2 v., Chicago, 1930) 1: pp. 506–507.

[4] John Burnet, *Early Greek Philosophy* (London and Edinburgh, 1892), p. 220.

history, took the prolongevitist vagaries of magic and folklore and fashioned them into a rationalized and disciplined system. Thousands of adepts studied and practiced that system and passed it on from generation to generation and from century to century. In the course of time, Taoist prolongevity techniques had a strong impact on Chinese science and medicine and also influenced, to some extent, Western science and medicine. It is for these reasons that Taoism must be given a leading position in the study of the development of ideas about the prolongation of life.

In order to appreciate Taoist ideas about prolongevity, it is necessary to have a grasp of the key events of Taoist history and the basic concepts and principles of Taoist ideology. Taoism is one of the two chief indigenous Chinese ways of thought (the other being Confucianism), and as such it has had a long and rich development.[5] The greater part of this chapter will be devoted to a review of Taoism in its three main aspects: philosophy, religion and "protoscience." Each will be considered in regard to its history, its characteristic ideas and especially its relationship to prolongevitism.

PHILOSOPHY [6]

To Westerners the most familiar aspect of Taoism is Taoist philosophy, particularly the teachings ascribed to Lao Tzu. These teachings, embodied in a treatise known as the *Tao Te Ching* (*The Classic of the Tao and its Power*), have been the cause of much controversy among sinologists.[7] The interpretation of the

Tao Te Ching is in doubt, its date of composition is in doubt, and even its authorship is in doubt, for, historically speaking, Lao Tzu is more a symbol than a real person.[8] What is not in doubt is that this brief and enigmatic work has exerted a tremendous influence in China and also has aroused considerable interest in the West, where it has appeared in more translations in English, for example, than any book except the Bible.[9]

The two other leading Taoist philosophers are Chuang Tzu and Lieh Tzu, whose writings usually are referred to simply as the *Chuang Tzu* and the *Lieh Tzu*. The *Chuang Tzu* differs in tone from the *Tao Te Ching*; it is much more direct and contentious and includes many commentaries and parables illustrating the tenets of Taoism.[10] The *Lieh Tzu* is a lesser work lacking either the jewel-like perfection of the *Tao Te Ching* or the eloquent versatility of the *Chuang Tzu*.[11]

It was in the period 350–250 B.C. that the three Taoist classics were written [12]; that makes them contemporary with the works of such Western philosophers as Aristotle and Epicurus. Although when they first appeared, they did not propound any explicitly religious teachings, over the years they were given more and more a theological slant by certain Taoists until finally in the period A.D. 150–200 an organized Taoist church sprang into existence. Other Taoists, however, preferred to carry on their speculations in a non-theological tradition. A current of philosophical Taoism runs through the entire course of Chinese history, exerting a strong influence not only in philosophy but also in art and literature.[13]

The significance of philosophical Taoism for this study is that its classical period provided the intellectual framework for ancient and medieval Chinese speculation about

[5] Two brief introductions to Taoism are Homer H. Dubs, "Taoism" in *China*, Harley F. MacNair, ed., United Nations Series (Berkeley, 1946), pp. 266–289 and J. J. L. Duyvendak, "Taoism" in *Encyclopedia of Social Sciences* (New York, 1934) 14: pp. 510–513. A study which is more profound (and more controversial) is Needham, "The *Tao Chia* (Taoists) and Taoism," *SCC* 2: pp. 33–164. The best history of Taoism (but poorly documented) in a Western language is Holmes Welch, *The Parting of the Way: Lao Tzu and the Taoist Movement* (Boston, 1957), pp. 88–163; this work hereafter will be referred to as "Welch, *Parting*." It may be supplemented by the well-annotated study by the same author, "Syncretism in the Early Taoist Movement," *Papers on China* (duplicated for private distribution by the East Asia Program of the Committee on Regional Studies, Harvard University) 10 (1956): pp. 1–54; this paper may be obtained on microfilm from the Harvard-Yenching Library. I wish to thank Prof. Benjamin Schwartz, the eminent sinologist, for reading this chapter and the next while they were in preparation.

[6] For an authoritative exposition of Taoist philosophy, see the relevant sections of Yu-lan Fung, *History of Chinese Philosophy*, Derk Bodde, transl. (2 v., Princeton, 1952). More spirited, and with a strong emphasis on ethics, is Welch, *Parting*, pp. 18–87. For the milieu of early Taoist philosophy, see Arthur Waley, *The Way and its Power: a Study of the "Tao Te Ching" and its Place in Chinese Thought* (Boston, 1935 and New York, 1958), pp. 17–100; this book hereafter will be referred to as "Waley, *Way*."

[7] A good standard translation is by James Legge in *The Texts of Taoism*, Sacred Books of the East (2 v., Oxford, 1891) 1: pp. 45–124; This work hereafter will be referred to as "Legge, *Texts*." A more poetic rendition which seeks to recapture the

original spirit of Lao Tzu is Waley, *Way*, pp. 141–243. An interesting contrast is provided by a translation (based on the commentary of an eighth-century Taoist) by Frederic Henry Balfour, *Taoist Texts: Ethical, Political and Speculative* (London and Shanghai, 1884), pp. 1–48.

[8] For a most lucid explanation of the controversies about Lao Tzu, see Welch, *Parting*, pp. 1–17.

[9] This statement is made by Welch, *Parting*, p. 4; he lists some thirty-five English translations which appeared between 1868 and 1955.

[10] For English translation, see Legge, *Texts* 1: pp. 127–392 and 2: pp. 1–232.

[11] Extensive selections are translated in Lionel Giles, *Taoist Teachings from the Book of "Lieh Tzu,"* Wisdom of the East Series (London, 1912). For the complete work, see the French translation in Léon Wieger, *Les Pères du système Taoiste* (Hsienhsien, 1913, and Paris, 1953), pp. 65–199 or the German translation by Richard Wilhelm, *Liä Dsi* (Jena, 1921).

[12] The extant version of the *Lieh Tzu* is believed to date from as late as the fifth century, but it contains much material from the earlier period; cf. Fung, *op. cit.* (see fn. 6) 2: p. 191.

[13] For the evolution of philosophical Taoism after A.D. 200, see Welch, *Parting*, pp. 123–126, 158–163; Fung, *op. cit.* (see fn. 6) 2: pp. 168–236, 407–433; and Needham, *SCC* 2: pp. 432–505. It is interesting to notice the frequent and respectful references to Taoist prolongevitism by the brilliant eighth-century poet Tu Fu; William Hung, *Tu Fu, China's Greatest Poet* (Cambridge, Mass., 1952).

prolongevity. While it is debatable whether Lao Tzu, Chuang Tzu, and Lieh Tzu themselves believed in the possibility or desirability of prolongevity, it is indisputable that most of their teachings readily could be interpreted in a way to support prolongevitism. And that is exactly what happened; the school of Taoist prolongevitism *adapted* the philosophical classics to serve the cause of prolongevity. This ideological heritage provided the means by which vague and random prolongevitist tendencies of primitive folklore were fashioned into a disciplined and respectable system.[14] Just how the three classics lent themselves to that sort of use will be analyzed as we pass in review the characteristic principles of philosophical Taoism.

UNITY OF NATURE

Taoist metaphysics centers on the word *tao* (pronounced "dow"), which means literally "the way." In a general sense the *tao* is nearly synonymous with Nature, especially with Nature conceived of as a process, so that the *tao* may be said to represent "the way" the universe works.[15] More specifically, the *tao* is the fundamental reality underlying the world of Nature; it is the changeless unity which exists behind the screen of apparent change and plurality.

. . . Dependent on nothing, unchanging,
All pervading, unfailing.
One may think of it as the mother of all things under
heaven.
Its true name we do not know;
"Way" is the by-name that we give it.[16]

All nature being a manifestation of a single force, the *tao*, the distinctions between various types of phenomena remained comparatively blurred. Particularly noteworthy was the lack of a sharp antithesis between mind and matter; Maspero has noted the significance of this for prolongevitism.

If the Taoists in their search for longevity, conceived it not as a spiritual but as a material immortality, it was not as a deliberate choice between different possible solutions but because for them it was the only possible solution. The Graeco-Roman world early adopted the habit of setting Spirit and Matter in opposition to one another . . . But the Chinese never separated Spirit and Matter, and for them the world was a continuum passing from the void at one end to the grossest matter at the other. . . .[17]

[14] This observation was made by Max Weber, *The Religion of China: Confucianism and Taoism,* Hans H. Gerth, transl. (Glenco, Illinois, 1951), p. 191. In general, Weber's studies of East Asian religions are far less productive than his famed work on the "Protestant Ethic."
[15] *Tao Te Ching,* chap. 34 in Waley, *Way,* p. 185.
[16] *Ibid.;* chap. 25, p. 174.
[17] Quoted and translated by Needham, *SCC* 2: p. 153, from Henri Maspero, *Le Taoisme* (Paris, 1950), p. 17. Maspero and Needham are somewhat puzzling in their use of the term "material" immortality when dealing with a pantheistic system in which little contrast was drawn between matter and spirit. I owe this observation to Prof. George D. Goldat.

The unity of nature also gave support to the concept of transformation, so important for alchemy. For example, Ko Hung, the greatest Taoist alchemist, argued that it was possible for animals to be changed from one species to another, for lead to be transformed into gold and for a human being to be converted into a *hsien* (an immortal being).[18]

PANTHEISM

The conception of the *tao* was so sweeping and all-pervading as to give it some of the attributes of a Godhead. According to Lao Tzu, "Tao alone supports all things and brings them to fulfillment" and "through it all things are done." [19] This omnipotence of the *tao* called forth a reverent attitude.[20] The wise man was he who yearned to come into communion with the *tao* and identify himself with its purposes: "the Sage clasps the Primal Unity, testing by it everything under heaven." [21] These ideas about the *tao* seem to fit the definition of pantheism as a doctrine in which the universe as a whole is God. But in Taoist philosophy the theological inclination never was made that explicit, and the best descriptive phrase available is the somewhat contradictory one used by Needham, "naturalistic pantheism." The importance of naturalistic pantheism for prolongevitism is that it tended to break down the division between man and the gods; each human being possessed a spark of the divine which was his by natural right to develop as he would.

MYSTICISM

Both the epistemology and the ethics of Taoism were characterized by mysticism. The *tao,* which above all things is worth knowing, is not accessible to the mind except through emotional insight. It cannot be heard or seen or expressed in words; [22] yet the highest goal of the sage is to contact it and understand it; this is accomplished by contemplation and trance leading to an ecstatic mystical experience.

"Just now, your body, Sir, was like the stump of a rotten tree. You looked as if you had no thought of anything, as if you had left the society of men, and were standing in the solitude (of yourself)." Lao Tan replied: "I was enjoying myself in thinking about the commencement of things. . . . The comprehension of this is the most admirable and the most enjoyable (of all acquisitions)." [23]

As we shall see, the techniques of achieving this emotional link-up with the *tao* were to be utilized as part of the process for attaining prolongevity.

[18] Ko Hung, *op. cit.* (see fn. 1), chap 2, pp. 141–144, 179–182.
[19] *Tao Te Ching,* chap. 37 and 41 in Waley, *Way,* pp. 188, 193.
[20] *Ibid.,* chap. 51, p. 205.
[21] *Ibid.,* chap. 22, p. 171.
[22] *Chuang Tzu,* book 22 in Legge, *Texts* 2: p. 69.
[23] *Ibid.,* book 21, 2: pp. 46–48. My discussion of mysticism and other features of philosophy and religion owes much to the classic, William James, *Varieties of Religious Experience.*

QUIETISM

Perhaps ecstasy is too strong a word for the mystical realization of the Taoist, for his precepts enjoined him to avoid passion and sensuality. The leitmotif of Taoist ethics was *wu wei,* best translated as "effortless action," [24] which ruled out aggressiveness, vivacity or purposefulness.[25] A large part of the classics is devoted to the idealization of quietism; the sage is pictured as seeking out the lowest level like water, playing a passive, almost feminine role in life, avoiding honors and riches and excessive learning.

PRIMITIVISM [26]

In social ethics, quietism expressed itself in ideas along the line of the Western adage: that government is best which governs least. But Taoist *laissez faire* was advocated not so that society might advance to greater wealth and complexity, but rather that it might return to the simplicity of olden times, the Chinese equivalent of the Age of Gold, when men lived modestly and naturally.[27]

PROLONGEVITISM

Each of these principles of classical Taoist philosophy lends itself to the idea that life may be greatly lengthened.[28] The unity of nature opens the possibility of transformation from a short-lived form of life to a long-lived one. Naturalistic pantheism endows man with a spark of the divine, which, without having any original sin to overcome, he may learn to increase by his own effort. Mysticism offers a means of communion with the vivifying power of the *tao.* Quietism provides a method of conserving one's vital forces, and primitivism teaches that man may recover the insights and way of life which allowed the sages of ancient times to attain prolongevity.

Primitivism furnished the means for integrating the prolongevity themes of Chinese folklore with the ideology of Taoist prolongevitism. The classics implied that miraculous powers were not merely within the range of possibility; they already had been possessed and used by the sages of the past. The "True Men of Old," as described by Chuang Tzu, "could ascend the loftiest heights without fear; they could pass through water without being made wet by it; they could go into fire without being burnt. . . ." [29] Later, Chuang Tzu speaks

of one of these ancient sages attaining the age of twelve hundred years without suffering the infirmities of bodily decay.[30] These passages not only merged smoothly with antediluvian and hyperborean-type legends [31] but also initiated the cult of the *hsien,* which had a central place in prolongevitist thought. The legendary material will be dealt with more fully later in this chapter and the idea of *hsien*-ship in chapter V.

The principle which could be interpreted most readily as endorsing the idea of prolongevity was quietism. Taoist ethical teachings imply that, if one wishes to live long, one should avoid the strife and struggle which are associated with ambitions for wealth and wordly fame.

> Heaven is eternal, the Earth everlasting.
> How come they to be so? It is because they do not
>   foster their own lives;
> That is why they live so long.
> Therefore the Sage
> Puts himself in the background. . . .[32]

Remarks of this kind frequently are met with in the writings of Lao Tzu and Chuang Tzu [33]; they are correlated with the postulate that man is born with a fixed amount of some vital substance, which is consumed either slowly or quickly according to his rate of activity.

> But to fill life to the brim is to invite [bad] omens.
> If the heart makes calls upon the life-breath, rigidity
>   follows.
> Whatever has a time of vigor also has a time of decay.[34]

Here the warning is made that the emotions (i.e., the heart) tend to use up the original supply of vital breath allotted to each individual.[35] The precept that temperance promotes longevity, particularly focal in Taoist quietism, is found throughout the history of geriatrics; we shall meet it again, for example, in the Renaissance work of Cornaro, *De vita sobria.*[36]

Oddly enough, the Taoist interpretation of quietism initiated a cult of skill which further enhanced the growth of prolongevitism. The central notion of Taoist quietism was not inactivity but rather "effortless action" (*wu wei*), an ideal exemplified by the ability of skilled craftsmen to achieve large results with a minimum of effort. Because the sage's actions were effortless, he was able to avoid depletion of his vitality, just as an experienced artisan is able to extend the life of his tools by using them cleverly. This moral was conveyed by Chuang Tzu in the words of a butcher whose ability was admired by the king:

"Observing the natural lines (my knife) slips through the great crevices and slides through the great cavities, taking

---

[24] Duyvendak, *op. cit.* (see fn. 5), p. 511.

[25] *Chuang Tzu,* book 15 in Legge, *Texts* 1: pp. 365–366.

[26] On the idea of primitivism, see earlier, chap. III.

[27] *Chuang Tzu,* book 9 in Legge, *Texts* 1: p. 278.

[28] Previous authors have neglected to investigate these ways in which Taoist prolongevitism was logically derived from the tenets of classical Taoist philosophy. What discussion there is has centered on the rather sterile controversy as to whether Lao Tzu and Chuang Tzu *themselves* believed in prolongevitism.

[29] *Chuang Tzu,* book 6 in Legge, *Texts* 1: p. 237.

[30] *Ibid.,* book 11, 1: p. 299.

[31] See earlier, chap. III.

[32] *Tao Te Ching,* chap. 7 in Waley, *Way,* p. 150.

[33] E.g., *ibid.,* chap. 15, p. 160 and chap. 52, p. 206 and *Chuang Tzu,* book 13 in Legge, *Texts* 1: p. 331.

[34] *Tao Te Ching,* chap. 55 in Waley, *Way,* p. 209.

[35] *Idem.,* "note 4." *Cf.* the lamp analogy of Avicenna, see earlier, chap. II.

[36] See later, chap. VII.

advantage of the facilities thus presented. My art avoids the membranous ligatures, and much more the great bones. . . . Now my knife has been in use for nineteen years; it has cut up several thousand oxen, and yet its edge is as sharp as if it had newly come from the whetstone. . . ." The ruler Wan-hui said, "Excellent! I have heard the words of my cook, and learned from them the nourishment of (our) life [i.e., the means to enhance one's vital forces]." [37]

While stories of this type pictured the prolongation of life by conserving one's vital energies, at the same time they opened up another path to prolongevity through the winning of skill in manipulating the forces of nature. Like the craftsman, the sage was envisioned as one whose knowledge gave him wonderful powers over nature, and the prolongevitist school of Taoism included among the powers of the sage (and later the *hsien*) the ability to lengthen life indefinitely.

The mysticism of the classics contributed to prolongevitism the idea that it was practicable to commune with the *tao* in such an intimate manner as to imbibe some of its divine attributes.

He who having used the outer-light can return to the inner light
Is thereby preserved from all harm.[38]

By putting himself in touch with the *tao,* the sage became both purified and strengthened.

What Tao plants cannot be plucked,
What Tao clasps cannot slip.
By its virtue alone can one generation after another carry on. . . .
Apply it to yourself and by its power you will be freed from dross.[39]

By being fraught with the power of the *tao,* one became immune to the attack of insects or wild animals, one's vital forces were heightened, one's bodily constituents acted in perfect harmony; one became rejuvenated.[40] With this, there is the inference that health and longevity are signs of grace.[41]

Thus, if there were not the Tao, the bodily form would not have life, and its life, without the attributes (of the Tao), would not be manifested. Is not he who preserves the body and gives the fullest development to the life, who establishes the attributes of the Tao and clearly displays It, possessed of kingly qualities? [42]

The literal interpretation of such passages gave sanction to Taoists of the prolongevitist persuasion.

It is fascinating to notice in Lao Tzu and Chuang Tzu a number of indications that the techniques of mysticism already were being accommodated to the goal of prolongevity. These techniques originally were intended

to bring about a state of trance or self-hypnosis which gave the sage a sense of mystical communication with the *tao*.[43] The physical methods, alluded to briefly in the classics, seemed to consist of staring fixedly and controlling the respiration.

The True men of old . . . Their breathing came deep and silently.
The breathing of the true man comes (even) from his heels,
While men generally breathe (only) from their throats.[44]

Waley aptly has compared the process with that of the yoga of India.[45] In addition to serving to initiate a trance-like ecstasy, such techniques occasionally are correlated with the miraculous powers of the sage. When asked how the sage is able to travel unharmed through fire and water and to penetrate to the secret knowledge of all things, the Taoist replies:

It is by his keeping of the pure breath (of life). . . .
By gathering his nature into a unity, by nourishing his vital power, by concentrating his virtue. . . .[46]

The state of trance is compared with the condition of early childhood, considered by Taoists to be the time of maximum health, and the manner of inducing the trance is termed "the regular method of guarding the life." [47] The *Tao Te Ching* speaks of the sage acquiring a strength that nothing can overcome:

This is called the art of making the roots strike deep by fencing the trunk, of making life long by fixed staring.[48]

Students of Taoism disagree as to whether these statements mean that prolongevitism already was entrenched in the teachings of Lao Tzu and Chuang Tzu. Maspero, for example, feels that prolongevity was a Taoist aspiration from the very first, while Welch argues forcefully against that interpretation.[49] For our purpose the debate is largely irrelevant. What is important, and at the same time indisputable, is that later Taoists adapted the words of the Fathers to justify a belief in the possibility of prolongevity and to indicate some of the means of winning it.

APOLOGISM

After the above analysis of the ways in which prolongevitism was derived from Taoist philosophy, it may come as a surprise to find that the classics themselves show leanings to apologism. In the *Tao Te Ching* we read that, "to leave the subject of living altogether out

---

[37] *Chuang Tzu,* book 3 in Legge, *Texts* 1: pp. 199–200.
[38] *Tao Te Ching,* chap. 52 in Waley, *Way,* p. 206.
[39] *Ibid.,* chap. 54, p. 208.
[40] *Ibid.,* chap. 55, p. 209.
[41] *Cf.* Old Testament and Calvinist ideas of this-worldly signs of divine grace.
[42] *Chuang Tzu,* book 12 in Legge, *Texts* 1: pp. 310–311.

[43] For a discussion of techniques used by the early Taoists to induce a trance, see Waley, *Way,* pp. 116–120.
[44] *Chuang Tzu,* book 6 in Legge, *Texts* 1: p. 238.
[45] See earlier, fn. 43. There is need for a comparative study of Taoist and Yoga techniques; *cf.* Needham, *SCC* 1: p. 153 and 2: p. 144, "note e."
[46] *Chuang Tzu,* book 19 in Legge, *Texts* 2: p. 13.
[47] *Ibid.,* book 23, 2: pp. 80–81.
[48] *Tao Te Ching,* chap. 59 in Waley, *Way,* p. 213.
[49] Maspero, *op. cit.* (see fn. 17), pp. 201–218 and Welch, *Parting,* pp. 91–95.

of view is better than to set a high value on it." [50] Such statements are infrequent and rather vague in the *Tao Te Ching,* but in the *Chuang Tzu* the apologist tone becomes unmistakable.

And Phang Zu [or P'eng Tzu] is the one man renowned to the present day for his length of life: if all men were (to wish) to match him, would they not be miserable? [51]

. . . the Superior man . . . rejoices not in long life, and grieves not for early death. [52]

Most telling of all is a passage in which Chuang Tzu ridicules techniques of respiration and nutrition as a means of prolonging life and contrasts such physical striving with the placidity and indifference of the sage. [53]

The fact is that the principles of classical Taoism lend themselves almost as readily to apologism as to prolongevitism. Quietism, for example, would seem to rule out both the ambition to live long and the effort required to reach such a goal.

The True men of old knew nothing of the love of life or of the hatred of death. Entrance into life occasioned them no joy; the exit from it awakened no resistance. Composedly they went and came. [54]

In addition to this, the principles of pantheism and the unity of nature led to a relativist view of death, which was subversive of prolongevitism. If there were no discontinuities in nature, how could one draw a sharp line between life and death? And if all natural phenomena, including death as well as life, were reflections of the divine *tao,* how could men distinguish one of them as good and condemn the other as bad?

Since death and life thus attend on each other, why should I account (either of) them an evil? . . . (Life) is accounted beautiful because it is spirit-like and wonderful, and death is accounted ugly because of its foetor and putridity. But the foetid and putrid is transformed again into the spirit-like and wonderful. . . . [55]

His [the sage's] distinction is in understanding that all things belong to the one treasury, and that death and life should be viewed in the same way. [56]

In keeping with this line of thought are Chuang Tzu's musings as to whether death might not be likened to an awakening from a dream. [57]

And yet, explicit as they may seem, these apologist tendencies did not preclude the development of the pro-

longevitist school of Taoism. For one thing, ancient Chinese scripts were so laconic and ambiguous as to allow very different interpretations to be made of the same passage. This vagueness of the texts accounts for contradictions in modern translations. Legge, for example, translates a line from the *Tao Te Ching* as, "all life-increasing arts to evil turn," which makes it seem an apologist statement. [58] Waley, however, renders the same line as, "to fill life to the brim is to invite omens," [59] thereby making it an admonition to practice moderation so that life may be prolonged. Most of the apologist expressions which follow from the principles of quietism can be considered as being aimed not at prolongevitism *per se* but at prolongevity techniques being practiced in an excessively narrow or active manner. All through the literature of Taoist prolongevitism there are warnings that physical methods alone are not sufficient for the attainment of immortality; that ethical and religious considerations also must enter into account. And the adepts also were advised time and again that they ought not to try to storm the heights but rather should carry on their exercises with quiet and patience. In this way the apparent apologism of the Fathers was adapted to the service of prolongevitism.

Similarly, many of those apologist statements which stemmed from relativism could be read as veiled references to a prolongevitist concept, "the deliverance of the corpse," according to which the successful adept might seem to die but in actuality had gained immortality. [60]

The ancients described (death) as the loosening of the cord on which God suspended (the life). What we can point to are the faggots that have been consumed; but the fire is transmitted (elsewhere), and we know not that it is over and ended. [61]

This statement, within the context of Chuang Tzu's thought, can best be understood in terms of pantheism; the divine spark is not lost at death but returns to the *tao* from whence it will issue again in some other form. But taken into the framework of prolongevitist concepts, the same statement might seem to refer to "the deliverance of the corpse" by a sage who, having transformed himself into a *hsien,* leaves behind a cadaver which is merely an empty husk. Another example is the paradoxical remark of Lao Tzu, "When one dies one is not lost, there is no other longevity." [62] This may be understood either in a broad pantheistic sense or in a more narrow prolongevitist one. In favor of the latter interpretation (in terms of "the deliverance of the corpse" concept), the prolongevitist might cite a further passage from Lao Tzu:

---

[50] *Tao Te Ching,* chap. 75 in Legge, *Texts* 1: p. 118.
[51] *Chuang Tzu,* book 1 in Legge, *Texts* 1: p. 167. On P'eng Tzu, see later, section on Chinese magic and folklore.
[52] *Ibid.,* book 12, 1: pp. 309–310.
[53] *Ibid.,* book 15, 1: pp. 364–365.
[54] *Ibid.,* book 6, 1: p. 238. This praise of serenity reminds one of Hellenistic Stoicism and Epicureanism; see earlier, chap. II.
[55] *Ibid.,* book 22, 2: p. 59.
[56] *Ibid.,* book 12, 1: p. 310.
[57] *Ibid.,* book 2, 1: pp. 194–195.

[58] *Tao Te Ching,* chap. 55 in Legge, *Texts* 1: p. 99.
[59] *Ibid.* in Waley, *Way,* p. 209.
[60] On the "deliverance of the corpse," see later, first section of chap. V. Cf. earlier chap. II, section on New Testament.
[61] *Chuang Tzu,* book 3 in Legge, *Texts* 1: pp. 201–202.
[62] *Tao Te Ching,* chap. 33 in Waley, *Way,* p. 184.

If, then, the Sage . . . when he has achieved his aim does not linger, it is because he does not wish to reveal himself as better than others.[63]

Thus, the apologism of the classics, so clear to some modern sinologists, did not present an insurmountable barrier to Taoist prolongevitism.[64]

RELIGION [65]

While Taoist philosophy contributed the intellectual framework for Chinese prolongevitism, Taoist religion provided the institutional forms and the fervent conviction necessary for the large-scale practice and transmission of prolongevity techniques. Before the appearance of the Taoist Church, some blending already had occurred between Chinese prolongevitist folklore and the teachings of Taoist philosophy. But that synthesis might not have been carried to fruition, and its results might have remained very circumscribed in space and time had it not been for the powerful impetus provided by the rise of a Taoist Church with its zealous drive for the salvation of its members from disease and death.

Classical Taoist philosophy, as we have seen, had certain religious proclivities; by 100 B.C., certain individuals identified with both Taoism and magic were paying homage to divinities who later figured prominently in the Taoist pantheon.[66] The model for institutionalizing such Taoist worship may have been set by Buddhism, which arrived from India about A.D. 65.[67]

Suddenly in A.D. 184 extensive areas of eastern China were swept by the rebellion of the "Yellow Turbans," a social movement which marks in spectacular fashion the emergence of the Taoist Church. The prophet of the new religion had been Chang Tao Ling, who had set up in Western China a Taoist organization which rose in revolt at the same time as the Yellow Turban uprising.[68] These movements represent in Chinese history the first mass religion of personal salvation; like Islam, it was a fighting creed which sought political and economic as well as theological authority. Some of the more remarkable features of the new faith were its high degree of organization, its policy of equality

for women, its fervent communal ceremonies of a revivalist nature, and its strong concern with health and longevity.[69] The military power of the rebel units was overcome slowly by the central government by about A.D. 214, but the Taoist ecclesiastical hierarchy maintained its existence.

Taoist religion reached its apogee of influence and creativity during the period A.D. 200–600.[70] A great many sacred works were written, not only commentaries on the classics but also records of divine revelations from heavenly visitations; these writings were collected in the Tao Tsang, the canon of Taoism, which came to include more than fourteen hundred treatises.[71] However, from A.D. 600 to 1100 the outward prestige and prosperity of the Taoist Church masked an inner decay. The bonds between the Taoist priesthood and its mass following became loosened; the less speculative drifted to a resurgent Confucianism, and the more religiously inclined joined the flood-tide of Buddhism. After 1200 Taoism was openly in decline; no outstanding priests or teachers appeared thereafter. The monks became more and more isolated and esoteric, while the lay priests tended to occupy themselves with exploiting the market for sorcery among the superstitious populace. In the twentieth century, religious Taoism has been moribund,[72] but the impact of Taoist notions still continues in the mores and folklore of the masses.

The Taoist Church was linked with currents of social and economic revolt; in that regard, it contrasted with the more conformist attitude of Confucianism and the other-worldly leanings of Buddhism.[73] The peculiar Taoist combination of practicality, popularity, and superstition also was expressed in the multitude of magical services rendered by the priests. In addition to teachings and charms designed to lengthen life, there were such practices as geomancy (the determining of the most propitious site for homes, tombs, etc.), exorcism (the expelling of evil spirits from the body, fields, etc.) and chronomancy (the deciding of lucky times for the performance of various acts).[74]

At first the priesthood diligently tried to lead all the faithful along the road to immortality; every member of

---

[63] Ibid., chap. 77, p. 237.

[64] There is an interesting passage in which the Taoist alchemist Ko Hung criticises Chuang Tzu's attitude towards death and directly attacks the apologist tendency *within* the Taoist movement; Ko Hung, Pao-p'u Tzu, Tenney L. Davis and Kuo-fu Ch'en, transl. in Proc. Amer. Acad. of Arts and Sciences 74 (1941) : pp. 307, 323.

[65] On Taoist religion and its history, see Needham, SCC 2: pp. 154–161; Welch, Parting, pp. 135–157; Weber, op. cit. (see fn. 14), pp. 173–219; J. J. M. De Groot, The Religion of the Chinese (New York, 1910), pp. 132–163 and Francis C. M. Wei, The Spirit of Chinese Culture (New York, 1947), pp. 128–154.

[66] Welch, Parting, pp. 99–103. There is much information about the early blending of folklore and magic with Taoist philosophy and religion in Yü, op. cit. (see fn. 2)

[67] Welch, Parting, pp. 118–119.

[68] Ibid., pp. 113–123 and Welch, "Syncretism" (see fn. 5), pp. 26–29.

[69] For the practices of the Taoist church in the epoch of the Yellow Turbans, see Maspero, op. cit. (see fn. 17), pp. 149–184.

[70] For the evolution of Taoist religion after A.D. 200, in addition to Needham and Welch, see Henri Maspero and Jean Escarra, Les Institutions de la Chine (Paris, 1952), pp. 63-69, 84-87, 105-107.

[71] These works are listed and described by Léon Wieger, Le Canon taoïste (Hsienhsien, 1913, and Paris, 1953).

[72] An account by one who visited China in 1948 is given by Wing-tsit Chan, Religious Trends in Modern China (New York, 1953), pp. 146–156.

[73] The radical socio-economic attitudes of Taoism are emphasized, perhaps overemphasized, in Needham, SCC 2: pp. 100–132.

[74] On the magic practices of the Taoist priests, see De Groot, op. cit. (see fn. 65), pp. 157–162 and Needham, SCC 2: pp. 346–364.

the church was required to perform prolongevity techniques to some degree, and the Taoist religion assumed the aspect of a gigantic health cult. In time, however, a gap began to open between those who were able to devote only a small part of their time to such practices and those able to follow them wholeheartedly. As the prolongevity techniques became more complicated and time-consuming, there arose a portentous distinction between the *adept* and the ordinary believer. Even the lay priests, concerned with their daily round of churchly activities, tended to lose contact with prolongevitism. The pursuit of immortality became more and more restricted to the monasteries, where it took on an esoteric and even symbolic character. The breakdown in communication between the adepts and the lay members can be identified as one of the main causes of the decadence and decline of religious Taoism.[75]

PROTO-SCIENCE

In addition to serving as inspiration for Taoist religion, the classics of philosophical Taoism also stimulated a large proportion of the scientific study and speculation of ancient and medieval China. This relationship between Taoism and science has been established by the painstaking analysis of Needham [76] which led him to the conclusion that,

The philosophy of Taoism . . . developed many of the most important features of the scientific attitude. . . . Moreover, the Taoists acted on their principles, and that is why we owe to them the beginning of chemistry, mineralogy, botany, zoology and pharmaceutics in East Asia. They show many parallels with the scientific pre-Socratic and Epicurean philosophers of Greece.[77]

The three aspects of Taoism which are related to science are naturalism, empiricism, and the cult of skill. If these attributes seem out of place in a mystical ideology like Taoism, one need only recall the honorable place in the history of science of the medieval Islamic "Brethren of Sincerity" movement or of Western figures like Bruno and van Helmont.[78] Such mystics, with their opposition to any sort of rigid scholastic rationalism, at times have sponsored a productive empirical approach to nature.

The term "proto-science" borrowed from Needham, is useful in suggesting that the scientific strands within Taoism represent science in its embryonic form rather

than its mature state. Taoist observation of nature was not systematic enough, and there was very little quantitative treatment of the data. There was too much respect for traditions handed down from the golden past and, at the same time, too much stress on spontaneity and intuition to allow objective interpretation of the data. Furthermore, the Taoists so mistrusted the sharply reasoned arguments of the Confucians that they never worked out the logical methods necessary for the precise definition of concepts and the orderly elaboration and testing of hypotheses. These shortcomings should be kept in mind when one deals with the "scientific" aspects of Taoism.

Taoist philosophy was naturalistic in the sense that it was intensely interested in natural phenomena, and also in that it did not provide for any divine power outside of the processes of nature. Naturalistic pantheism endowed nature itself with a holy quality, and the Taoist, therefore, regarded natural phenomena with a mixture of reverence and keen curiosity. The influence of naturalistic pantheism accounts for many of the sensitive observations and interpretations of natural events which are found in Taoist writings. The empiricism of Taoist proto-science was enhanced by quietism. Shunning the city and the court, the Taoist, like Thoreau, sought out a retreat, where he might watch with a tranquil mind the workings of natural forces. He rejected any attempt to impose on natural phenomena a distinction between "good" and "bad." Asked where the *tao* might be found, Chuang Tzu replied: everywhere—in the ants, in weeds, in brick and tile and even in dung.[79] Here was scientific insight similar to that expressed in Aristotle's dictum that *all* nature is wonderful (i.e., worthy of careful study).[80]

Taoist proto-science was saved from passivity by the cult of skill which runs through the classical works. The ideal of *wu wei* or "effortless action," as we have seen, was envisioned as a sort of jiu jitsu with which the sage, through his insight into natural processes, was able to achieve great results with the smallest expenditure of energy. The admiring stories of the skill of craftsmen formed a link between philosophy and technology, a relationship which proved fruitful in the inception of an experimental method in Chinese science. At the same time, the Taoist cult of skill is a forerunner of the Baconian view (see later, chap. VIII) that science is the means for bringing nature into the service of man; this may be seen in a thirteenth-century commentary on a Taoist alchemical treatise.

I would say that man as he exists in the universe is merely a thing in that universe. Yet because his spirituality is greater than that of other creatures, he is given the special name of "man." How, then, can he stand co-equal

---

[75] Maspero and Escarra, *op. cit.* (see fn. 70), pp. 85–86.

[76] Needham, *SCC* 2: pp. 33–164 and 442–452. Needham's work on the scientific aspect of Taoism was anticipated, in a limited way, by Fung, *op. cit.* (see fn. 6) 2: pp. 431–433. Needham, at times, carries to extreme lengths his theses that science, democracy and socialism are essential for each other and that Taoism represents a forerunner of all three.

[77] Needham, *SCC* 2: p. 161.

[78] *Ibid.* 2: pp. 89–98. Allen G. Debus has been producing a series of studies explaining the role of mystics in early modern Western science, most effectively in "Robert Fludd and the Use of Gilbert's *De Magnete* in the Weapon-Salve Controversy," *Jour. Hist. Medicine and Allied Sciences* 19 (1964): pp. 389–417.

[79] *Chuang Tzu*, book 22 in Legge, *Texts* 2: p. 66.

[80] Quoted (from *On the Parts of Animals*, I, 5) on the frontispiece of Charles Singer, *History of Biology* (New York, 1950).

with Heaven and Earth? If he seize for himself the secret forces of Heaven and Earth, in order thereby to compound for himself the great elixir of the golden fluid, he will then exist coeval with Heaven and Earth from beginning to end. Such a one is called the True Man.[81]

In this regard, Taoism manifests, as Yu-lan Fung has noted, one of the essential aspects of science, the striving for power over nature.[82]

The strongest stimulus for Taoist proto-science was the desire to extend decisively the length of life. If Taoism was instrumental in initiating in China certain parts of the sciences of chemistry, biology, and medicine, it is largely because these fields of study were directly concerned with the prolongation of life. The Taoists entered the domain of physiology, when they attempted to devise beneficial breathing practices and physical exercises. They carried out pioneer work in chemistry and botany, because they were seeking drugs with vivifying properties. Clearly, Taoist empiricism and the cult of skill were harnessed to serve the elaboration of prolongevity techniques.[83]

MAGIC AND FOLKLORE

Although ancient Chinese records are too ambiguous and incomplete to allow firm conclusions about priority, the evidence indicates that magic and folklore in China, as elsewhere, antedated philosophy. It seems safe to assert, that, at the time the *Tao Te Ching* first was written down, there already were in existence legends which inculcated the desirability and possibility of greatly increasing the life span, and there were being followed various magic rites which aimed at reaching that goal.

As in folklore in other parts of the world (see earlier, chap. III), one of the basic concepts in Chinese prolongevity legends was the antediluvian theme, that the length of life had been much greater in the past. A much-revered personage in that regard was P'eng Tzu, who, according to folklore, lived more than eight hundred years, during which time he served as a high official for the earliest emperors.[84] P'eng Tzu did not die even then but disappeared into the western mountains; he may be considered the personification of longevity and has been termed the Taoist Methuselah. Unlike Methuselah, however, P'eng Tzu was not the longest-lived of the ancients, for he had received instruction from Pai Shih, who retained the appearance of a man of forty but had reached the age of nearly three

thousand years. The antediluvian theme harmonized with the primitivism of Taoist philosophy; we already have found Chuang Tzu speaking of one of the sages of yore who enjoyed twelve hundred years of earthly existence. Chinese prolongevity traditions of the antediluvian type also strengthened the Taoist concept of *hsien*-ship which will be described in the next chapter.

A second influence on Taoist prolongevitism came from legends of the hyperborean type, that the life span is much greater in certain parts of the world. There were several Chinese versions of the hyperborean theme, the most compelling of which were the accounts of the Isles of the Eastern Sea,

These three divine (island) mountains were reported to be in the Sea of Po, not so distant from human (habitations), but the difficulty was that when they were almost reached, boats were blown away from them by the wind. Perhaps some succeeded in reaching (these islands). (At any rate, according to report) many immortals (*hsien*) live there, and the drug which will prevent death is found there.[85]

These were the words of the early Chinese historian Ssu-ma Ch'ien; a similar description of the isles may be found in the Taoist classic the *Lieh Tzu*.[86] Also in the *Lieh Tzu* is the story of another paradise, this one far in the north like the Hyperborean land of Greek tradition. In "Northendland" the span of life was fixed at exactly one hundred years, and during that time the marvelous waters of the place prevented any disease or aging.[87] A third land of longevity was believed to be in the distant west in the realm of the mythical queen Hsi Wang-mu, whose garden produced miraculous peaches with the property of conferring immortality.[88] As in Western Europe, these hyperborean legends stimulated exploration,[89] the most famous expedition being the one sent out to search for the Isles of the Eastern Sea in 219 B.C. by Ch'in Shih Huang Ti, the emperor who first unified China and built the Great Wall.[90] Such legends being taken literally, the prolongevitist bent in Taoism was strengthened, and these lands of folklore were adapted to serve as the abode of Taoist *hsien*.

Chinese folklore also included the third basic type of prolongevity legend characterized by what we have termed the fountain theme, the idea that there exist various substances with the quality of prolonging life.

---

[81] Fung, *op. cit.* (see fn. 6) 2: p. 432.

[82] *Ibid.*, "The Scientific Spirit of Religious Taoism," 2: pp. 431–433. *Cf.* the optimism of Jabir, see later, chap. VI, section on Arabic alchemy.

[83] For the physiological techniques, see later, chap. V. For the alchemical techniques, see chap. VI.

[84] On P'eng Tzu, see such standard reference works as Herbert A. Giles, *A Chinese Biographical Dictionary* (London and Shanghai, 1898), p. 624 and E. T. C. Werner, *A Dictionary of Chinese Mythology* (Shanghai, 1932), pp. 431–432.

[85] Quoted (from the *Shih Chi*, 28: 10b–11b) in Needham, *SCC* 2: p. 240.

[86] *Lieh Tzu*, chap. 5 in Wieger, *op. cit.* (see fn. 11), pp. 131–133.

[87] *Ibid.*, chap. 5, p. 137.

[88] Obed S. Johnson, *A Study of Chinese Alchemy* (Shanghai, 1928), p. 60 and Giles, *op. cit.* (see fn. 84), p. 272.

[89] The role of hyperborean legends in Chinese expansion to Japan and Central Asia was noted by Weber, *op. cit.* (see fn. 14), p. 197.

[90] Welch, *Parting*, pp. 97–98. On the abode of Hsi Wang-mu in the Kunlun Mountains, the immortality cult at the Han imperial court, and the resulting geographical expansion, see Yü, *op. cit.* (see fn. 2).

The prototype for the theme in Western culture is the story of the fountain of youth, in which certain waters were alleged to have miraculous properties. The same idea occurs in the Chinese "Northendland" where senility was prevented by the waters of the "Divine Spring."

The perfume of the water was more delicious than that of orchids or pepper, and its taste was better than that of wine or ale. . . . The people were gentle . . . they lived in joy and bliss . . . having no decay and old age. . . . They bathed and swam in the waters, and on coming out their skins were smooth and well-complexioned. . . .[91]

Chinese tradition also spoke of wonderful fruits with youth-preserving effects, for example the peaches of immortality in the western paradise of Hsi Wang-mu and the fruit, mentioned in some accounts of the Isles of the Eastern Sea, which conferred immunity from both old age and death.[92] Still more significant was the version which located on the eastern isles "the drug which will prevent death," for it reveals an early tie between prolongevitism and pharmaceutics. These fountain-type legends meshed with and influenced Taoist prolongevitism, particularly its dietary and alchemical techniques.

Especially noteworthy in Chinese prolongevity legend is a rather minor theme of other cultures, the phoenix theme, which ascribes to certain animals an exceedingly long life span. According to Chinese nature lore, there were a number of exceptionally long-lived animals, most notable of which were the tortoise and the crane, each reported to live over a thousand years.[93] The "fact" that species other than man attained such grand longevities was cited by Taoist prolongevitists in replying to sceptics; the alchemist Ko Hung, for example, often used this line of reasoning.[94] Some of the Taoist prolongevity techniques were supposed to be patterned on the breathing and dietary practices of the crane and tortoise, and, similarly, the ingestion of such foods as crane's eggs and tortoise soup was held to be life-prolonging.[95] Pines and cypresses also were believed to exist a millennium or more, and products of these trees, therefore, were valued as ingredients of prolongevity medicaments.[96]

The evidence indicates that the origin of Taoist prolongevitism owed much to the activities of the shamans and magicians of ancient China.[97] For one thing, there is the similarity in the trance-like state sought by both the shamans and the Taoists. The Taoist interpreted the experience in terms of communion with the *tao*, but he used the same symbolism as the shamans. Also alike was the preoccupation of both groups with magic controls over nature; like the shamans, the Taoist priests were practitioners of exorcism, divination, weather control, healing, etc., and the *hsien* were deemed especially potent in such matters.[98] Most telling of all is the evidence that, already in early times, the shamans were concerned with the prolongation of life: several ancient shamanist songs have been preserved which are dedicated to the god of longevity (later highly regarded in religious Taoism),[99] and an early work on geography mentions shamans who have discovered death-banishing herbs.[100]

CONCLUSION

We now may summarize the probable origins of Taoist prolongevitism by saying that prolongevity legends and techniques already existed in China before the advent of Lao Tzu and Chuang Tzu, and that this rather amorphous prolongevitism drew ideological justification from classical Taoist philosophy and was given institutional backbone by Taoist religion. In return, it is likely that Taoist philosophy and religion received wider popularity because of their association with the prolongation of life. Having passed in review the chief components which entered into its genesis, we now turn to an investigation of Taoist prolongevitism as it flourished, fully-formed, in the period A.D. 300–1000.

V. TAOIST PROLONGEVITISM IN PRACTICE

Taoist prolongevitism held two complementary aspirations: the ultimate goal was immortality, the more immediate one was the prolongation of life. Faced with the fact that life is short but art is long, the adept had a powerful motivation for trying to lengthen his years so as to enhance his chances of earning eternal life. While involved in the time-consuming search for an elixir of immortality, the adept might sustain his powers by taking drugs of lesser purity and potency.[1]

. . . some drugs are better than others . . . the vegetable drugs . . . enable one to cure diseases, to rectify shortcomings, to preserve juvenility, to do without cereal food, and to strengthen the breath, although they can not confer actual immortality. At the best, they will prolong life for a few hundred years, in other cases they will only fortify the natural constitution, and can not be relied upon for long.[2]

[91] *Lieh Tzu*, chap. 5, quoted by Needham, *SCC* 2: p. 142.
[92] *Ibid.*, chap. 5 in Wieger, *op. cit.* (see fn. 11), p. 133.
[93] Ko Hung, *op. cit.* (see fn. 1), pp. 184–186.
[94] *Ibid.*, pp. 183–193. Cf. the similar reasoning by Peter Martyr, see earlier, chap. III, fountain theme.
[95] *Ibid.*, pp. 181, 189, 191–193 and Johnson, *op. cit.* (see fn. 88), pp. 61–62.
[96] Ko Hung, *op. cit.* (see fn. 1), pp. 184–186, 198.
[97] For a summary of the data associating Taoism with shamanism and magic, see Needham, *SCC* 2: pp. 132–139 and Mircea Eliade, *Le Chamanisme* (Paris, 1951), pp. 393–395.

[98] On the powers of the *hsien*, see later, chap. V.
[99] Arthur Waley, *The Nine Songs: a Study of Shamanism in Ancient China* (London, 1955), pp. 37–43.
[100] Needham, *SCC* 2: pp. 135–136.
[1] Ko Hung, *Pao-p'u Tzu*, chap. 4, Eugene Feifel, transl., *Monumenta Serica* (Peking) 9 (1944): pp. 5–6.
[2] Ko Hung, *Biographies of "Hsien,"* "Liu Ken" in Lionel Giles, *A Gallery of Chinese Immortals*, Wisdom of the East Series (London, 1948), pp. 58–59. The work by Giles hereafter will be referred to as "Giles, *Immortals.*"

Similar to the range of results from drugs were the varying effects of the physiological and ethical practices which brought one increasing longevity according to the quantity and quality of one's efforts. An illustrative story is that of a certain Wang Chen, who began Taoist studies at the age of seventy-nine; after some thirty years of diligent practice (i.e., at the age of 109), he was able to restore his appearance to that of a young man of thirty, but it was not until several hundred years later that he finally became an immortal (*hsien*).[3]

THE "HSIEN"

The *hsien* or immortals were men who had won eternal life by means of their mastery of the techniques of prolongevity.[4] In Western culture there is nothing exactly comparable to a *hsien*; he might be thought of as combining some of the traits of saint, angel, and sage. Like a saint, the *hsien,* at least partly due to his piety and morality, was venerated as a holy person by a religious movement. But he differed from the saint in that his distinction was based to a great extent on skill in the abstruse arts, his nature often was rather gay and capricious, and there was no formal process for his beatification. The *hsien* was similar to an angel in having a status much higher than that of ordinary men yet lower than that of the gods, whom he served as a sort of messenger and aide-de-camp. However, the *hsien* was not pictured angel-fashion as a paragon of beauty and grace but rather as a gnarled, shrewd-looking fellow.[5] A *hsien* held the qualities of knowledge and wisdom which characterize a sage, but while the sage clearly remained a human being, the *hsien* had transformed himself into a higher being.

The *hsien* had all sorts of marvelous powers at his command: he could control the weather, travel at incredible speed, assume the appearance of various animals or make himself invisible. All this is reminiscent of the descriptions, probably symbolic, in the *Tao Te Ching* and the *Chuang Tzu* of the attributes of the "Sages" and the "True Men of Old."[6] There were three different realms which the *hsien* might choose as his dwelling place; he might live on earth among ordinary men, he might travel to one of the terrestrial paradises like the Isles of the Eastern Sea, or he might rise to heaven itself. In general, the celestial or heavenly *hsien* were considered the most successful and meritorious, but there was a strong this-worldly bias in Taoism, and it

was recognized that some *hsien* might prefer terrestrial existence. It was said of Po Shih Sheng, who retained his youth at an age of more than two millennia,

He had no longing to ascend on high, but aspired to nothing more than a long life on earth. . . . When somebody asked him why he did not wish to fly up to heaven, he replied: "I'm not at all sure I should enjoy myself as much in heaven as I do in this world."[7]

The lives and exploits of the *hsien* were the subject of an extensive and colorful literature.[8] The earliest collection dates from the third century; one of the best was compiled a century later by Ko Hung, the great alchemist. To give the flavor of the latter work, we may quote briefly from the life of Chang Tao-ling, the founder of the Taoist Church.

He began as a student at the Imperial Academy, and made a thorough study of the Five Canonical Books. "Alas!" he exclaimed with a sigh, "all this study will not add to my span of life"; so he set himself to master the principles of longevity. . . . In course of time Chang Tao-ling amassed much treasure wherewith to buy the drugs he needed in order to compound the elixir. When the elixir was ready, however, he only took half a dose, for he did not want to rise up to heaven immediately.[9]

The taste for miracles led to more elaborate versions, and, in a much later account, the story of Chang Tao-ling ended on a magnificent note.

At noontide the whole host of *hsien* formed round him a guard of honor, and to the strains of celestial music escorted him to the topmost peak of the Tower-in-the-Clouds Mountain. Thus at the age of 123 the Saintly One ascended to heaven in broad daylight.[10]

The *hsien* legends also dealt with women as well as men.[11]

Only a few of the greatest saints were able to reach immortality like Chang Tao-ling in the full glare of public attention; the vast majority of adepts had to undergo a more modest form of apotheosis known as the "deliverance of the corpse." This process involved the *apparent* death and burial of the sage. To unbelievers it would appear that illness and death had carried away another ordinary mortal; but those initiated into the secrets of Taoist lore would realize that the supposed corpse represented only a sword or a piece of bamboo which the successful adept had caused to assume human form so as to mask his attainment of *hsien*-ship.[12]

---

[3] *Ibid.,* "Wang Chen," p. 69.

[4] On the *hsien,* see Giles, *Immortals,* pp. 7–14 and Joseph Needham, *Science and Civilization in China* (Cambridge, 1954ff.) 2: pp. 139–143, 152–154. The work by Needham hereafter will be referred to as "Needham, *SCC.*"

[5] *Hsien* often are pictured in traditional Chinese painting; examples of the gnomelike appearance can be seen in Laurence Sickman and Alexander Soper, *The Art and Architecture of China,* Pelican History of Art (Harmondsworth and Baltimore, 1956), plates 91B and 130.

[6] See earlier, chap. IV.

[7] Huan-ch'u, "Po Shih Sheng" in Giles, *Immortals,* p. 18. On the evolution of the concept of the *hsien* from an other-worldly to a this-worldly one, see Ying-shih Yü, "Life and Immortality in the Mind of Han China," *Harvard Jour. Asiatic Studies* 25 (1964–1965): pp. 80–122.

[8] On the *hsien* literature, see Needham, *SCC* 2: pp. 152–153.

[9] Ko Hung, *op. cit.* (see fn. 2), "Chang Tao-ling," pp. 60–61.

[10] Huan-ch'u, "Chang Tao-ling" in Giles, *Immortals,* p. 64. This account was written a thousand years later than the one by Ko Hung.

[11] E.g., "Mao Nü" in Giles, *Immortals,* p. 35.

[12] For the classical sanction for the "deliverance of the corpse" idea, see earlier, chap. IV, section on Taoist philosophy.

The better way of obtaining release from the flesh is by means of a sword; the inferior method is by means of bamboo or wood. Dipping your brush into the divine elixir, you write on the sword blade the charm of the Supreme Mystic Yin Sheng, and in a little while the sword is transformed into the shape and appearance of the person who is being translated, and lies quietly on the bed while the real man disappears.[13]

To substantiate this explanation, stories were told of the reappearance of *hsien* after their "death" and burial, and how, when the coffin was disinterred, the cadaver no longer could be found.[14]

Ch'ang-fang said: "What you buried long ago was only a bamboo stick." Thereupon they dug up the grave and broke open the coffin, and, sure enough, found the stick still inside.[15]

The "deliverance of the corpse" was only the last scene in a long drama of internal transformation.[16] By following prolongevity practices over many years, the adept felt that he was changing his body, bit by bit, to a more subtle and pure material. His tissues became analogous to the most rare and imperishable matter; his bones became as gold, his flesh as jade. Finally, when the interior evolution was completed, he became a *hsien* and abandoned his old body which had become merely a dried-up hollow shell like the cocoon of a metamorphosed butterfly. While the "deliverance of the corpse" was compared to the metamorphosis of insects, the internal transformation of the body was thought to be similar to the development of the human embryo. The prolongevity techniques themselves were termed "imitation of the embryo," for it was believed that the adept, like an embryo in the womb, was able to carry on gaseous exchange without breathing and to take in nourishment without eating.[17] And the *hsien* was like a new-born infant, which, according to Lao Tzu, was a stage of life immune to injury, with the bodily harmony at its most perfect and the vital force at its height.[18]

We now are prepared to examine the actual techniques of Taoist prolongevitism. The four major physiological techniques were the respiratory, dietary, gymnastic, and sexual. As they are described, it should be kept in mind that they were practiced simultaneously without any sharp distinction being drawn between them. Also, it must be remembered that these proto-scientific endeavors took place in an aura of religious speculation, and, in order to make that more apparent, a fifth type of practice will be analyzed, the "spiritual" techniques. Finally, there is a sixth type, the alchemical techniques, which will be examined in the next chapter.

RESPIRATORY TECHNIQUES [19, 20]

Among the physiological practices of the Taoists, the cardinal place was reserved for breathing techniques. That was because, in Taoist cosmology, the breath was a link between the human and the divine.[21] Man was thought of as a sort of mixture of earth and air; earth was the more impure, gross, and inert, while air was more pure, subtle, and active.[22] Air was identified with the spirit and thence with the divine; the air around us blended with the sky which, in turn, bordered on heaven. Some of this reminds one of the ideas of the Greeks, who, in their physiology, also emphasized respiration and, in their cosmology, also viewed the heavens as the realm of eternal and godlike qualities. But while the Greeks postulated a sharp division between the terrestrial (including air) and the celestial spheres, the more pantheistic outlook of the Taoists allowed a much greater degree of intermingling. Therefore, to the Taoists the possibility arose that, if one regulated one's respiration correctly, one might make intimate physical contact with the heavenly realms, and gain, thereby, the immortality of the gods.

The respiratory techniques must be understood within the conceptual scheme of microcosm and macrocosm, according to which man (the microcosm) and the world (the macrocosm) operate in a similar manner and have many attributes in common. The world, for example, was thought of as an enormous organism which carried on respiration like any other living being. During the night the macrocosm breathed out (expiration), and the

---

[13] "Pao Ching" in Giles, *Immortals,* p. 105.

[14] Here the deliverance narratives are parallel to Christian accounts of the Resurrection; Matthew 28 and Mark 16. Cf. earlier, chap. II, section on New Testament.

[15] Huan-ch'u, "Fei Ch'ang-fang" in Giles, *Immortals,* p. 81.

[16] On the internal transformation into a *hsien,* see Henri Maspero, "Les Procédés de 'nourrir le principe vital' dans la religion taoiste ancienne," *Jour. asiatique* 229 (1937): pp. 180–182.

[17] The embryo, of course, receives its oxygen and nourishment from the mother via the blood vessels of the placenta and umbilical cord.

[18] *Tao Te Ching,* chap. 55 in Arthur Waley, transl., *The Way and its Power* (Boston, 1935 and New York, 1958), p. 209. This idealization of early life correlates with the social primitivism of Taoism. A somewhat similar combination of views is found in the West in Rousseau; e.g., *The Social Contract* and *Émile.*

[19] By far the best accounts of the physiological techniques are the brilliant studies of the Taoist canon, the *Tao Tsang,* by Henri Maspero in the *Jour. asiatique* (see fn. 16), supplemented by Henri Maspero, *Le Taoisme* (Paris, 1950), pp. 15–24, 83–116. These works hereafter will be referred to as "Maspero, *JA*" and "Maspero, *Taoisme.*" In English, there are useful but brief reports (based largely on Maspero) by Needham, *SCC* 2: pp. 139–152, and Holmes Welch, *The Parting of the Way: Lao Tzu and the Taoist Movement* (Boston, 1957), pp. 105–112, 120–121, 130–135. The book by Welch hereafter will be referred to as "Welch, *Parting.*"

[20] On the respiratory techniques, see Maspero, *JA,* pp. 197–252, 353–378 and *Taoisme,* pp. 107–114; Needham, *SCC* 2, pp. 143–144 and Welch, *Parting,* pp. 108–110, 130, 132.

[21] It was common in early thought to associate breath, life, soul and God; cf. the Greek word *psyche* which, at first, meant breath and later came to mean soul; also there is the statement in the Old Testament that after God had formed man from dust, He "breathed into his nostrils the breath of life, and man became a living soul"; see Charles Singer, *A History of Biology* (rev. ed., New York, 1950), pp. 15–16.

[22] Maspero, *Taoisme,* pp. 113–114.

night, therefore, was known as the period of dead breath when the atmosphere was saturated with expired air. The time of "living breath" was during the day, when the macrocosm breathed in (inspiration). The Taoist adept practiced his respiratory exercises at the time he considered a period of living breath; in most cases, this was during the daylight hours.[23] There was, however, a good bit of variety; many felt, for example, that the air reached its high point of salubrity just before dawn as it started to warm and just at sunset as it started to cool. An opposing school of thought, disturbed by the fact that the times of sunrise and sunset vary throughout the year, argued that the hour of the exercises should be determined "by the clock"; from noon to midnight was the period of dead breath, while the period of living breath was from midnight to noon.

The preparations for the exercises were guided by tediously ritualistic formulas regarding not only the optimum time of day but also location, position, prayers, and ablutions. Such details varied markedly among different schools of prolongevity. A typical procedure, however, might be as follows:[24] Fast for a period long enough to allow all excrement to be eliminated from the body. Wash yourself carefully; then retire to a large quiet room which has been freshly whitewashed and is furnished in a very simple manner. Purify the room by burning incense, seat yourself on a mat and meditate on the precepts of Taoism. After grinding your teeth several dozen times (to intimidate evil spirits) and carrying out a number of long expirations to rid the body of impure breath, you are ready to begin. Preparations of this sort illustrate the aura of magic and religion which was never absent from Taoist prolongevity activities.

The long-term goal of the adept was to be able to gain enough nourishment from the air, a pure spirit-like material, that he might dispense with the ingestion of grains (rice, wheat, etc.), which, being the products of earth, were believed to have a deleterious effect on the body.[25] To draw increased sustenance from the air, three difficult skills had to be acquired: first, the adept had to learn to retain the breath much longer than in normal breathing; second, to guide the breath to parts of the body not regularly accessible to it; and third, as the breath was about to be expired, to catch it in the throat and swallow it. The entire procedure was known as "embryonic respiration," for it was believed to be similar to the respiration of the embryo in the womb.[26]

Those who follow the *tao*, if they desire to master Embryonic Respiration . . . must . . . breathe as the fetus in the abdomen breathes; that is why these exercises are termed Embryonic Respiration. In coming back to the

roots, in returning to the origin, one overcomes old age and comes back to the condition of the fetus.[27]

Thus, the adept sought "nourishment by the breath" in order to gain the perfect bodily harmony which Lao Tzu had ascribed to the newborn.

Of the three skills leading to "embryonic respiration," the most arduous to develop was the first: the retention of breath.[28] Such practices began easily enough with holding the breath for a period of time equal to three, five, seven, and nine normal respirations; on reaching twelve, one was said to have completed a "small series." From there the way was more difficult, for it was necessary to add one small series to another until the retention of breath covered a time equal to one hundred twenty normal respirations; this constituted a "large series," and it was from this point on that the procedure was considered to exert a major benefit on one's health. Most writers urged the adept to carry on his daily exercises until he approached at least two large series; even then his ultimate goal remained distant, for immortality became possible only when the breath could be retained for one thousand respirations.

The adepts were encouraged by the appearance of symptoms which we would ascribe to lack of oxygen (anoxia), but which they attributed to successful manipulation of the breath.[29] When hands and feet tingled and the face became flushed, the adept felt that he had been able to pervade those body parts with unusually large and beneficial amounts of breath.[30] When he achieved the lightheadedness and carefree feeling (euphoria) which accompany anoxia, he must have believed that his body, being freed of its earthier qualities, was taking on the ethereal nature of the *hsien*.[31] At the same time that he gave this optimistic interpretation to the anoxic syndrome, the adept also was aware of the hazards involved.

. . . after a time equal to three hundred respirations, the ears no longer hear, the eyes no longer see and the heart no longer thinks[32]; then it is necessary little by little to cease retaining the air.[33]

---

[23] On the question of the optimum time for respiratory exercises, see Maspero, *JA*, pp. 355–361.

[24] *Ibid.*, pp. 354–362.

[25] Maspero, *Taoisme*, pp. 112–113.

[26] See fn. 17.

[27] *Tao Tsang* in Maspero, *JA*, p. 198. As only a few of the more than fourteen hundred treatises of the Taoist canon have been translated into any Western language, quotations will be cited under the general term *Tao Tsang;* data regarding treatise, chapter, and page number may be obtained in Maspero's footnotes. These quotations represent translations by Maspero from Chinese to French and by myself from French to English. Words within brackets are my own additions.

[28] On the retention of breath, see Maspero, *JA*, pp. 203–206 and *Taoisme*, pp. 111–112.

[29] This was noted by Needham, *SCC* 2: p. 144.

[30] Maspero, *JA*, p. 205.

[31] Euphoria and loss of judgment are well-known hazards to pilots flying at high altitude and, therefore, subject to anoxia.

[32] It is common in early science to consider thinking a function of the heart rather than the brain: Herophilus (*ca.* 300 B.C.) is noted for recognizing the brain as the site of intelligence; Aristotle had placed it in the heart; *cf.* Arturo Castiglioni, *A History of Medicine*, E. B. Krumbhaar, transl. and ed. (2nd ed., New York, 1947), p. 185.

[33] *Tao Tsang* in Maspero, *JA*, pp. 204–205.

It is interesting to consider briefly these breath-retention exercises in the light of modern physiology. It might seem fantastic, at first glance, that the adept should be able to avoid breathing for a period equal to one hundred twenty respirations; however, a number of factors were operating to bring this within the range of possibility. For one thing, the rate of respiration is very variable, and, by timing their endeavors in this manner, the Taoists opened the way for erroneous calculations. If, for example, the retentions were being timed according to the breathing of an observer, as often was done, it is likely that, as the excitement mounted, the observer's respiratory rate would increase more and more. In cases where the time was left to be gauged by the adept himself according to his own conception of the normal rate of breathing, there was still greater likelihood of subjective distortion. But, even if we assume that the procedure were accurately timed, at least some of the goals might be attainable. Modern experiments show that, after training, certain persons can hold their breath as long as four and a third minutes [34]; if we figure twenty respirations per minute, the upper limit of relaxed respiration, then this would amount to about eighty-seven respirations. The necessary training methods involve strengthening the will and building up the lung's capacity to hold air (and consequently oxygen); also helpful is preliminary "overbreathing" to decrease the amount of carbon dioxide in the body. All of these factors could have been utilized by the adepts. In addition, it should be kept in mind that the adepts were subsisting on a near-starvation diet and were practicing an almost trancelike quietism. Therefore, the body metabolism of the adept would be quite low, and, his use of oxygen also being low, he might be able to maintain consciousness for five or six minutes (one hundred to one hundred twenty respirations).[35]

The guidance of the breath, the second stage of "embryonic respiration," reflects the usual Taoist mixture of traditional teaching, empirical observation and mystical speculation. In the view of traditional Chinese anatomy and physiology, the breath traveled the following route through the five body organs:[36] on inspiration, the breath was drawn into the nose and carried to the spleen, from which it descended to the liver and kidneys; on expiration, the breath was drawn back into the spleen, mounted from there to the heart and lungs and was expelled via the mouth. This path which the breath

traversed in ordinary persons missed, according to Taoist prolongevity thought, some of the most vital areas of the body, in particular the lower and upper "fields of cinnabar." These "fields of cinnabar" were pictured as small boxlike organs which, because of their strategic location and function, were vaguely analogous to cinnabar, the key substance in Chinese alchemy.[37] The existence of a lower field of cinnabar, located in the abdomen, seems to have been suggested by the sound of gases rumbling through the intestines, a phenomenon which was favored by the air-swallowing practiced by the adepts. The upper field of cinnabar, located in the center of the head, seems to be related to the spaces within the brain which today are termed the cerebral ventricles.

To divert the breath from its usual channels and send it to the fields of cinnabar, the adept employed a mystical device known as "interior vision." [38] By mental concentration he brought before his mind's eye a complete view of the interior of his body; then, by a combination of faith, prayer, and will power, he sought to direct the breath wherever he desired. The most difficult part was to get the breath from the spleen into the lower field of cinnabar, for, not only was the passage blocked by physical obstacles, it also was guarded by several divinities. It might take from ten months to three years to unlock the crucial entryway, but the effort was willingly made, because success meant the restoration of the respiratory circulation of the embryo.[39] Once within the lower field of cinnabar, just below the navel, the breath blended with the "essence" of the body, a vital liquid identified with the spermatic fluid. The potent mixture then was guided from the lower field of cinnabar to a passageway along the backbone which led to the upper field of cinnabar. There in the brain the concoction of breath and essence exerted a restorative effect, and then the breath passed down to the heart (the middle field of cinnabar), the lungs and finally the throat.

When the breath had returned to the throat, it was possible for the adept to advance to the third stage of embryonic respiration, "nourishment by the breath." [40] From time to time, instead of allowing the breath to pass from the throat to the mouth and be expired, the adept swallowed a mouthful of saliva in such a way as to trap the breath and bear it down into the stomach. This act was facilitated by the fact that, throughout the period of respiratory exercises, the adept kept his mouth filled with saliva (the so-called "broth of jade") in order to prevent air from entering the mouth (a happening which was accounted highly injurious). By bringing

---

[34] J. S. Haldane and J. G. Priestley, *Respiration* (New Haven, 1935), p. 181.

[35] The amount of oxygen needed by the body varies directly with the metabolic rate; for example, a patient's B.M.R. (basal metabolic rate) is measured by determining the amount of oxygen he takes in during a standard period of time. In surgery, cooling the body is employed to decrease the metabolic rate and to lower the need for oxygen when respiration or circulation is depressed. Also, see later, chap. VIII, on "anabiosis."

[36] Maspero, *JA*, pp. 182–185.

[37] *Ibid.*, pp. 191–197. On cinnabar in alchemy, see later, chap. VI.

[38] On the guidance of the breath, see Maspero, *JA*, pp. 212–246 and *Taoisme*, pp. 110–111.

[39] Maspero, *Taoisme*, p. 21.

[40] *Ibid.*, pp. 112–114.

the breath to the stomach, the prolongevitists believed they could nourish themselves without having recourse to ordinary foods, for, according to Taoist theory, the body was nourished by a process in the stomach which extracted an essence or breath from foods and sent that "food-breath" to the various organs. Whereas the food-breath from grains (rice, wheat, etc.) was relatively gross and impure, the air-breath was light and pure and heavenlike. That is why the adept, as much as possible, abstained from cereal foods and swallowed his breath; in so far as the food-breath was replaced by air-breath, he felt that he took on more and more the ethereal qualities of an immortal *hsien*.

Such were the respiratory techniques as they were practiced in the first several centuries of Taoist prolongevitism; later, in the T'ang period (*ca.* 600–900), the entire procedure was given a new slant by the elaboration of the doctrine of the "inner" breath.[41] The respiratory exercises which have been described were concerned with the manipulation of air from the atmosphere, and, in dealing with this "external" breath, the adept had been brought into contact with the outside world. But as Taoism, under the influence of Buddhism, became more contemplative and more inward, the idea gained currency that the external breath was of little account, and that the important factor in prolongevity was an "inner" breath given by the gods at birth to each individual.[42] Accordingly, the aim of most prolongevitists from the T'ang dynasty on was the conservation of this inner or "original" breath.

The principle is to absorb the Original Breath and to spread it among the viscera; when one succeeds in conserving the [inner] breath for a long time, one will not die. Why concern oneself with the external world and try to absorb the external breath?[43]

The inner (or original) breath was considered a vital principle located in the fields of cinnabar and identified to some degree with the saliva and the spermatic fluid. The adept, therefore, zealously sought to prevent the loss of these fluids and also labored to keep the inner breath from being carried away with the expired external breath. It was said that one was born with six "inches" of inner breath; if one prevented some of the usual losses, one's life would be lengthened significantly, and, if one retained the original six inches intact, one would live forever.[44]

All breathing exercises now were modified in line

with the new emphasis on the inner breath. The preparatory rituals became more diverse than ever, since the choice of time and place no longer had to accord with concepts of the macrocosm (external breath) but only with the personal whims of the adept himself (inner breath). The practice of retaining the breath was abandoned except in certain cases of illness. The guidance and swallowing of the breath were maintained, but with the important difference that it now was inner rather than external breath that was being directed through the body; therefore, swallowing now preceded guidance instead of following it. And guidance was elaborated by the addition of a new skill known as "melting" the breath which brought about some of the desirable symptoms previously associated with retaining the breath.[45] While abstaining from breathing, the adept allowed the inner breath to wander at will through the body; after some time, he experienced a feeling of warmth accompanied by profuse perspiration, symptoms which signified the achievement of a state of "melting." The procedure was highly esteemed because it was more passive than guiding the breath, and also because it seemed to be analogous to the alchemical "melting" or refining of cinnabar.

Before leaving the subject of breath, there should be mentioned a minor technique, interesting because of its anticipation of modern sun-bathing. In absorbing the "breath" of the sun, the simplest method was to face the rising sun and, after gazing at it for some time, to close the eyes and meditate on a spectrum of colors flowing from the sun to one's own body.[46] By mental power this spectrum was brought into the mouth and swallowed. The procedure was repeated forty-five times. The more advanced adept sought to capture not merely the colors but the image of the sun: holding in his left hand a picture of a red sun on a green background, he faced the sun until he saw an image of it the size of a large coin. By meditation, this replica of the sun was guided to the heart where it produced warmth and luminescence. The image then was passed out with the expired air, or, if the adept were more ambitious, it might be guided first to other parts of the body. The absorption of the sun's "breath" represents one more Taoist fusion of empiricism with mysticism, the inspiration, in this case, being the observation of the colorful after-images which appear when one closes one's eyes after looking at the sun.[47] Also there may have been some notice of the beneficial effects resulting from the exposure of the body to the sun. In this regard, the female adepts were at a distinct disadvantage, for their efforts were directed to the absorption of breath not from the sun but from the moon.

[41] On the "inner" breath school, see Maspero, *JA,* pp. 206–231.

[42] This reminds one of the "innate moisture" of ancient and medieval gerontology; as the innate moisture was used up, the body became senescent (cold and dry); see earlier, chap. II, section on biology and medicine.

[43] *Tao Tsang* in Maspero, *JA,* p. 227.

[44] Maspero, *JA,* p. 209. *Cf.* Cornaro's conservation of "inner moisture"; see later, chap. VII.

[45] On "melting" the breath, see *ibid.,* p. 219.

[46] On absorbing "breath" from the sun, see *ibid.,* pp. 374–377 and Needham, *SCC* 2: p. 145.

[47] Noted by Maspero, *JA,* p. 375.

DIETARY TECHNIQUES [48]

Intimately allied with the respiratory techniques were those practices concerned with diet. While the adept sought to control his breathing so that he might obtain more sustenance from the air, at the same time he tried to regulate his diet so as to decrease his intake of food, especially cereal (grainy) food. His long-range purpose here was to live on air and saliva and to avoid, thereby, the formation of bodily excrements which were regarded as emblems of impurity and mortality. In this rigorous course not only were grains prohibited but also meat, wine, and many vegetables. Only one meal was scheduled for each day and that, as much as possible, was to consist of such relatively beneficial items as roots, berries, and other fruit. It is not surprising that the accomplishment of such a regimen demanded the frequent use of medicines.

A touch of drama was added to the dietary procedures by the concept of an enemy within which had to be starved and drugged into submission. This inner foe was envisioned as the "Three Worms," malevolent beings which, from their strategic positions within the fields of cinnabar, worked for the destruction of the individual. Like the "original sin" of Christianity and the "death instinct" of Freudianism, the concept of the Three Worms served to explain those internal conflicts and shortcomings which hinder the perfectability of man. To them was ascribed the cause of apathy and melancholy and unworthy desires, for they profited from the sins of their host. Wishing for his early demise so that they might be freed from their bodily prison, the Three Worms were pictured as keeping a careful account of misdeeds, which they regularly reported to heaven to persuade the gods to decrease the life span of the host. The occurrence of disquieting dreams was explained as due to the battles which sometimes erupted between the subversive Three Worms and the loyal body divinities. Further, these demons directly brought about illness and aging, by attacking the vital centers: the "blue" worm in the upper field of cinnabar caused baldness, blindness, and deafness, the "white" worm in the middle field of cinnabar brought about diseases of the heart and lungs, while, in the lower field of cinnabar, the "red" worm stirred up intestinal disorders and arthritis.

The perfidious Three Worms also were blamed for creating an appetite for the five grains. These cereals (rice, millet, wheat, oats, and beans) were disliked partly because of the observation that carbohydrates tend to produce intestinal gases and flatus.[49] But the more basic reason was that grain was so closely identified with earth, an element prone to corruption and decay.

Grain is the essence of the earth; its agreeable taste is a snare created by evil demons. Its odor troubles the body spirits, and embryonic respiration fails; the spirits become bewildered and dejected.[50]

It is grain which is responsible, in the first place, for the existence of the Three Worms: while the embryo is forming inside the womb, the mother is eating grain, the "breath" of which pervades the newly conceived child and forms within it the Three Worms. No wonder the adepts looked on the five grains with dread.

The five cereals are the scissors which cut down life, they destroy the vital organs, they shorten the life span. If grain enters your mouth, do not hope for eternal life! If you desire to escape death, your intestines must be free of them![51]

To the anoxic symptoms caused by breath retention, there was added now the burden of malnutrition; for not only were grains prohibited but also meats, wine, and strong vegetables (e.g., onions), all of which gave off odors offensive to the body spirits. Such stringency brought about dizziness, weakness, fatigue, and intestinal disorders. Therefore, it was necessary to allow a transition of thirty or forty days during which the adept was permitted to ingest a finely ground flour. Also available to him were a variety of traditional Chinese tonics (prepared according to secret Taoist recipes) which were believed to kill the Three Worms: cinnamon, licorice, ginseng, sesame, etc.[52] With the aid of these expedients, the adept had to press himself forward to a meagre diet based on unusual substances endowed with life-giving qualities.

These prolongevity foods are a significant link between legend and proto-science; for they represent a rationalized version of the fountain theme, that there exist certain substances with the property of lengthening life. This theme, as has been seen, repeatedly appears in the world's folklore in such forms as the water of the fountain of youth, the intoxicating beverage of the soma plant or the marvelous fruit of the Isles of the Eastern Sea.[53] Taoist proto-science was able to adapt and use the idea, because it fitted in with the tendency of Taoist pantheism to give a vitalist interpretation not only to the phenomena of biology but also to those of chemistry.[54] The same vital principle or "essence," which, stemming from the divine *tao*, caused the manifestations of life, was to be found also in varying degree in every substance in the world. And when these substances were ingested, their store of vital principle was available to strengthen the essence of the person who had eaten them. Since the length of life was determined by the quality and quantity of one's essence, it was imperative

---

[48] The only good source on dietary techniques is Maspero, *Taoisme*, pp. 98–107.

[49] Maspero, *JA*, p. 204.

[50] *Tao Tsang* in Maspero, *Taoisme*, p. 101.

[51] *Ibid.*, p. 100.

[52] For typical recipes, see Maspero, *Taoisme*, pp. 103–105.

[53] On the fountain theme, see earlier, chap. III.

[54] This interpretation is inescapable to anyone studying Taoist prolongevitism; *cf.* Obed S. Johnson, *A Study of Chinese Alchemy* (Shanghai, 1928), pp. 56–58. Also see later, chap. VI.

for the adept to identify those substances richest in pure, spiritlike essence and to make them the basis of his diet.

To supplement the adept's intake of air and saliva, there was a host of vitalized materials of animal, vegetable or mineral origin. These prolongevity foods or "*hsien* medicines" were chosen for a variety of reasons.[55] Many of the organic products were singled out in accord with the phoenix theme, that there are plants and animals enjoying a much greater life span than that of man [56]: included here would be items like tortoise broth, crane eggs, and pine resin. Eggs of all sorts were valued in line with the Taoist regard for the perfect vitality of the embryo. Peaches were associated with the fruit in the Western Paradise of Hsi Wang-mu. Great numbers of herbs and minerals were venerated for such properties as a red color (like cinnabar), a resemblance to man or an animal (e.g., various roots), a slippery fluidlike texture or a translucent, glowing appearance. At the top of the list were such valuable minerals as pearls, mica, jade, silver, gold, and cinnabar. But the subject of *hsien* medicines, at this point, becomes so closely related to alchemy that further discussion will be reserved to the next chapter.

GYMNASTIC TECHNIQUES [57]

Taoist gymnastics are the only portion of their physiological program which definitely is known to have influenced Western medicine.[58] The setting for this transmission was, not surprisingly, the cosmopolitan and encyclopedic culture of eighteenth-century Europe. In 1779 a Jesuit missionary in China, J. J. M. Amiot, published a well-illustrated article on "Cong-fou" (*kung fu*), as the Taoist system of physical exercise was called at the time.[59] After outlining the methods and some of the rationale of *kung fu*, he expressed the following wish:

. . . the purpose of this article is not to teach *Cong-fou*, but to propose to physicians that they examine without prejudice a matter which is thought-provoking. If the theory which supports it is false, they may replace it with one more correct. Should there result from this some ideas valuable to humanity, we shall consider ourselves

well recompensed for our temerity in bringing out this article.[60]

Father Amiot's hope was well founded, for his treatise was studied carefully by Per Henrik Ling, the founder of Swedish medical gymnastics.[61] Ling's institute in Stockholm in the first half of the nineteenth century was one of the major centers in creating modern physical education, physiotherapy, and rehabilitation, and the system propounded by Ling and his students was a combination of Greco-Roman practices and the Chinese *kung-fu*.

In the Taoist regimen, the chief function of gymnastics was to aid the carrying out of the respiratory and sexual techniques. Having noticed the invigorating effect of exercise and the improved circulation which resulted from it, the Taoists evolved a theory of hygiene which stressed the part played by "obstructions" within the body as a cause of illness. These blockages hindered the circulation of the breath; therefore, when the adept practiced the retention and guidance of the breath, it was important that he accompany the procedure with suitable physical exercises designed to overcome any obstruction. Not only did gymnastics allow the breath to reach parts of the body which might otherwise have been inaccessible, but it also speeded up the whole process of breath-circulation, a factor which was valuable because the amount of time one can retain one's breath is so limited. Similarly, in the sexual techniques it was desirable that obstructions be eliminated so that the "essence" might travel to all parts of the body.[62] It was quite standard for a period of rhythmic physical exercise to be scheduled between every two breath retentions or between every two rounds of sexual intercourse. All this does not mean that gymnastics was limited completely to a supplementary role; to some extent it was honored as an independent means of prolongevity, for by keeping the body supple and by expelling harmful "breaths," it prevented disease and lengthened life.

Although there were a number of alternative schools of Taoist gymnastics, their differences were not profound, and by quoting from one of them we may gain an idea of a typical procedure. It should be kept in mind that for the adept performing these exercises the normal position was squatting on his heels (see the illustrations).

First, cross the hands above the head and draw them down to the ground. Carry out five respirations and then stop. This fills the stomach with air. . . .

Next, with your left hand touching your left knee, raise your right hand as high as possible. Then, with your right hand touching your right knee, raise your left hand as high as possible. Carry out five respirations, then stop. This expands the breath which is inside the abdomen. . . .

---

[55] On the *hsien* medicines, see Ko Hung, *op. cit.* (see fn. 1), chap. 11 in 11 (1946): pp. 1–32.

[56] In the case of certain trees, this idea was correct. On the phoenix theme, see earlier, chap. III, section on miscellaneous themes and chap. IV, section on magic and folklore.

[57] The best sources on the gymnastic techniques are Maspero, *JA*, pp. 413–427 and *Taoisme*, pp. 115–116. Useful for its bibliographical material and for data regarding Taoist influence on Western medical gymnastics is Needham, *SCC* 2: pp. 145–146. A study which is detailed and profusely illustrated but based on late texts and uneven in interpretation is John Dudgeon, "Kung-fu, or Medical Gymnastics," *Jour. Peking Oriental Society* 3 (1895): pp. 341–565.

[58] Alchemy is not included here with the "physiological" techniques.

[59] J. J. M. Amiot, "Notice du cong-fou" in *Mémoires concernant l'histoire, les sciences, etc., des Chinois; par les missionaires de Pe-kin* (Paris) 4 (1779): pp. 441–451.

[60] *Ibid.*, p. 451; my translation.

[61] On Ling, see Castiglioni, *op. cit.* (see fn. 32), p. 898. For the Taoist influence on Ling, see Marcelle Peillon, "Gymnastique et massages" in *Histoire générale de la médecine*, M. Laignel-Lavastine, ed. (3 v., Paris, 1938–1948) 3 (1948): pp. 638–639.

[62] On the "essence," see later, section on sexual techniques.

more this is done the more marvelous are the results. (Figure 4)

Link your hands and, with the "hook" formed thereby, take hold of the feet. Twelve times. Then return to the normal position. (Figure 8) [64]

These exercises were carried on in a rhythmical manner. Some emphasized movements of the limbs, others of the trunk; some included massage and others were carried out while the adept suspended himself from a rope. In certain cases the movements were supposed to imitate those of long-lived animals, such as the tortoise. At all times, the primary purposes remained the same: to aid the circulation of the breath and "essence," to overcome "obstructions" and to expel harmful breaths.

SEXUAL TECHNIQUES [65]

The enemies of the Taoists accused them of sexual promiscuity; while there was some substance to these charges, they were basically incorrect. In reality, the adepts considered casual and indiscriminate intercourse to be an exceedingly serious fault, because such practices caused an irremediable loss of the life-sustaining *ching* (essence or sperm). Each act of coitus of the ordinary kind decreased one's span of life. On the other hand, unlike the Buddhists, the Taoists sharply criticized sexual abstention, which they regarded as abnormal and unhealthy.

Man does not want to be without woman; if he is without woman, he becomes agitated; if he becomes agitated, his spirits become fatigued; if his spirits become fatigued, his longevity is decreased. . . . When one strives to retain the essence [by abstention], it is difficult to conserve it and easy to lose it, because one lets it escape, the urine becomes troubled and one is carried away by the illness of succubus [sexual dreams].[66]

The Taoists worked out a compromise by which they sought to avoid the malign results associated with both indulgence and abstention. It was a compromise which allowed, and even encouraged, sexual activity but at the same time placed controls on the nature of that activity.

We do not struggle against the natural tendency of man, and [yet] we are able to obtain an increase in longevity. Is that not pleasant? [67]

The purpose of the sexual techniques was twofold: to increase the *ching* and to conserve the *ching*. The augmentation of the *ching* (or essence) involved the frequent practice of *coitus reservatus:* i.e, the adept's partner would be brought to orgasm, but the adept himself avoided the completion of the sexual act. In this way it was believed that the adept had gained a sexual emanation or "breath" from his partner and thereby had

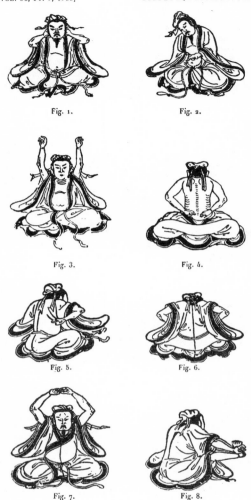

Fig. 1.

Fig. 2.

Fig. 3.

Fig. 4.

Fig. 5.

Fig. 6.

Fig. 7.

Fig. 8.

Next, cross your hands below your waist and turn rapidly right and left until tired. That makes the blood penetrate [more effectively] the vessels.   .

Next, cross your hands above your head and turn slowly right and left. This expands the breath inside the lungs and liver. . . .[63]

Here are several typical procedures described in the treatise which supplied our pictorial illustrations.

Bend the celestial column [the neck] to the right and left, thirty-six times in each direction. (Figure 2)

Massage the Hall of the Kidneys [area of back just below the ribs] with the hands, thirty-six times. The

[63] *Tao Tsang* in Maspero, *JA,* pp. 416–417.

[64] *Ibid.,* pp. 419–421.
[65] On the sexual techniques, see Maspero, *JA,* pp. 379–413 and *Taoisme,* pp. 114–115; Needham, *SCC* 2: pp. 146–152.
[66] *Tao Tsang* in Maspero, *JA,* p. 382.
[67] *Idem.*

strengthened his own *ching*. The process was considered nearly the opposite of the usual type of intercourse in which the penis entered in a large and firm condition and, after orgasm, became weak and flaccid; here the attempt was made to insert the penis in as languid a condition as possible and to finish the act with it strong and erect. In ordinary intercourse something was lost; here, it was believed, something must have been gained. Although it is simpler to describe the hypothesis in terms of the male adept, similar techniques might also be employed by a female adept to increase her own *ching*. Since it was most advantageous that the partner be brought to orgasm, the male and female adepts were not suitable for each other but had to find sexual associates outside the Taoist community.

What was this *ching* or essence which had so important a part in the prolongation of life? In the male it was identified with the semen; in the female, with the menstrual fluid. This does not mean these fluids were identical with the *ching;* they simply happened to be the most readily observable substances associated with it. The *ching* itself, while corporeal in nature, was something very subtle and ethereal.[68] Having observed that the semen and menstrual fluid become scanty in the ill and disappear in the "aged" (menopause and climacteric), it was quite reasonable for the Taoists to assume that longevity was proportional to the quantity and quality of the *ching*. But Taoist speculation was not content to rest with that deduction; the *ching* also was given the quality of revivifying the tissues of the brain, and, still more, the *ching* mixing with the breath formed, as from an embryo, that immortal body of the *hsien* which was liberated at the time of the "deliverance of the corpse."

Essence and breath unite and give birth to the Mysterious Embryo. The Mysterious Embryo establishes itself and gives birth to a body. That is the procedure of the Interior Cinnabar which allows one to escape death.[69]

The *ching*, therefore, not only was necessary for long life but also was the raw material for the attainment of immortality.

Carrying to its logical conclusion their hypothesis about increasing the *ching*, the adepts were led to the advocacy of an intensive program of sexual activity.

He who is able to have coitus several tens of times in a single day and night without allowing his essence to escape will be cured of all maladies and will have his longevity extended. If he changes his woman several times, the advantage is greater; if in one night he changes his partner ten times, that is supremely excellent.[70]

It was recommended that the partner be between fourteen and nineteen years old; in any case a woman over thirty was to be avoided if possible and one over forty was prohibited absolutely. While the woman ought to be young, she did not have to be particularly attractive so long as she was free of certain defects which were objectionable on physiological rather than aesthetic grounds: thick skin, masculine voice, certain body odors, hairy legs, and coolness of the body. As if to prevent the abuses inherent in such a system of sexual relations, the Taoists hedged about the entire proceeding with all sorts of other restrictions. For example, the period of intercourse had to be preceded by serious meditation and prayer, the body had to be clean, and one was not allowed to indulge in food or liquor. The most troublesome taboos had to do with time; these were so numerous that in any one year there were excluded at least two hundred days and in some systems even more.[71]

When the *ching* had been sufficiently aroused and increased by *coitus reservatus* with a succession of partners, it became necessary for the adept to allow himself to come to orgasm in such a way that the essence might yet be conserved; this practice was known as "making the *ching* return to repair the brain."

. . . when it [the *ching*] is about to be discharged, one quickly grasps with the two middle fingers of the left hand [the urethra] between the scrotum and the anus, one squeezes tightly while expelling from the mouth a long breath, at the same time grinding the teeth several tens of times.[72]

In terms of modern anatomy, this means that the semen was diverted to the bladder, from which it later would be excreted in the urine; similar procedures are used by various peoples for contraceptive purposes.[73] The adept, however, felt that the *ching* truly had been conserved, and that it was stored in the lower field of cinnabar. There it could be blended with the breath to form a highly potent rejuvenating substance which might be directed by "interior vision" to the brain and other parts of the body.

If you practice according to this rule, breaths and humors will circulate like a cloud, the fluid of the essence will be coagulated; whether you be young or old you will become as an adolescent. . . . If one practices (this procedure) a very long time, one becomes spontaneously a True Man and lives eternally through the centuries.[74]

What particularly scandalized the Buddhists and Confucians was the collective ritual known as "uniting the *yin* (female principle) and the *yang* (male principle)," a ceremony which involved sexual relations between the

---

[68] All this reminds one of the Aristotelian tradition (see earlier, chap. II) in embryology. Avicenna, for example, stated that the embryo is generated by the "innate heat," an ethereal substance in the semen, and the "innate moisture," a highly subtle fraction of the menstrual fluid; see O. C. Gruner, *A Treatise on the Canon of Medicine of Avicenna* (London, 1930), pp. 70–71, 100, 112, 114.

[69] *Tao Tsang* in Maspero, *Taoisme*, p. 115.

[70] *Ibid.*, in Maspero, *JA*, pp. 384–385.

[71] On the taboos regarding time, see Maspero, *JA*, pp. 397–400.

[72] *Tao Tsang* in Maspero, *JA*, p. 385.

[73] E.g., the Turks, Armenians and Marquesan Islanders; Needham, *SCC* 2: p. 149.

[74] *Tao Tsang* in Maspero, *JA*, pp. 386–387. After abstinence, the semen, of course, does appear thicker and "coagulated."

men and women of a church group apparently without regard to social status or family ties.[75] The practice seems to have arisen during the religious fervor and social upheaval which attended the establishment of the Taoist church in the second century. At the time of the new moon and again at the time of the full moon, all the adult believers (except unmarried girls) would assemble indoors, probably in small groups, to carry out the ritual. The procedure was strongly laden with religious meaning: there was an initial period of fasting for three days, there was a priestly instructor in control, and the avowed purpose was to deliver the faithful from their sins. As in so many of the practices of the early Taoist church, there seems here to be an attempt to act out, in a gross and naive manner, principles which Lao Tzu probably meant to be highly abstract; in this case, the ideas that the *yin* and the *yang* are both necessary to the world, and that their union is beneficial. At the same time, these collective sexual relations were connected, at least in part, with prolongevitist efforts to increase and conserve the *ching*: in ancient writings on the subject there is mention of the lower field of cinnabar, the need to prevent ejaculation and the goal of lengthening life.[76] Unfortunately, the descriptions from Taoist sources are fragmentary and vague, while those from Buddhist sources are prejudiced; therefore, it has not been possible to gain a clear picture of the matter.

As Buddhism made inroads into Chinese thought, and as Taoism became more mystical, the sexual techniques were more and more restricted, but they never were suppressed completely. Hardest hit, of course, were the collective rites: already in A.D. 415, one of the Taoist religious leaders had a vision in which a divinity ordered him to cleanse the church of the "false" practice of the union of *yin* and *yang*,[77] and by the seventh century, the sexual fetes had disappeared. The private procedures continued, though under an increasing veil of secrecy. "This procedure is absolutely secret: transmit it only to sages."[78] Even these techniques came under attack as some of the Taoist monasteries adopted the rule of celibacy; in the twelfth century, for example, one proponent of the new morality argued that the canonical passages dealing with sexual intercourse ought to be understood in an allegorical sense. By that time, however, the attitude of the Taoist church was irrelevant, for the sexual techniques had been taken up by secular Chinese and Japanese medicine and popular hygiene where they continued to be practiced even in recent years.[79]

SPIRITUAL TECHNIQUES [80]

To keep things in proper perspective, it may be useful here to give a short résumé of those Taoist religious practices which had a direct bearing on the prolongation of life. Despite the secular sound of many of the physiological techniques, Taoist prolongevitism was carried on in a religious milieu. The adepts believed that physical manipulations alone were not sufficient for prolongevity; it also was essential for one to follow a life of holiness.

He who aspires after immortality should, above all, regard as his main duties: loyalty, filial piety, friendship, obedience, goodness, fidelity. If one does not lead a virtuous life but exercises himself only in magical tricks, he can by no means attain long life.[81]

Thus the "material" transformation of the body into a divine substance is accompanied by a moral transformation. Here we find a similarity to Christianity, which seeks salvation not only from death but also from sin; as the eminent theologian John Baillie wrote, "the Christian tradition has not been interested in that [prolongation of life] as such, but in the hope for a totally new *quality* of life [italics his]."[82] This Christian tradition is not so different from many schools of prolongevity: the Taoists too, as we see, desired a new quality of life (freedom from sin and communion with the divine). Even in modern secular prolongevity, although the idea of communion with God is greatly decreased, there persists the idea that man will become "godlike."[83] And ethical perfectability remains a prominent feature; in Condorcet, moral improvement receives nearly as much attention as prolongevity, and in Godwin, even more.[84]

The Taoists developed the usual religious apparatus of prayer and veneration directed toward winning favor with the deities. These deities were extremely numerous; there were the thousands of divinities within the body itself (microcosm), and there was the hierarchy of divinities of the outside world (macrocosm). Through the practice of spiritual techniques one sought to appease this supernatural host and to win communion with higher and higher divine beings until ultimately one might reach a final apotheosis in mystical union with the *tao*.

The techniques directed towards the gods of the body (microcosm) consisted of a mixture of religious supplication and magical coercion. The gods within the body had a tendency to leave, and, therefore, one had to

---

[75] On the collective sexual rites, see Maspero, *JA*, pp. 400–409 and Needham, *SCC* 2: pp. 150–152.

[76] See the account by Chen Luan, a sixth-century Buddhist convert from Taoism; in Maspero, *JA*, pp. 404–405.

[77] Maspero, *JA*, p. 411.

[78] *Tao Tsang* in Maspero, *JA*, p. 386.

[79] On the recent practice of the sexual techniques, see Needham, *SCC* 2: p. 147, "note c."

[80] On the spiritual techniques, see Maspero, *Taoisme*, pp. 25–41, 85–89.

[81] Ko Hung, *op. cit.* (see fn. 1), chap. 3 in 6 (1941): pp. 209–210. These virtues are in contrast to the teachings of Lao Tzu and show the influence of Confucian ideas on Ko Hung.

[82] Letter to the author; 2-19-1957.

[83] E.g., Wynnewood Reade, *The Martyrdom of Man* (New York, 1874), pp. 512 ff. *Cf.* the remarks later about Stephens, Fedorov, and Leroux in chap. VIII, conclusion.

[84] On Condorcet and Godwin, see later, chap. VIII.

make a consistent effort to retain them, for their presence was essential to life. The complexity of the problem is suggested by the fact that there were some thirty-six thousand body divinities; each part of the body had one or more resident gods: there were four in the liver, six in the lungs, seven in the kidneys, etc. Most important of all were the gods in the "fields of cinnabar" controlling the head, chest, and abdomen.

The first step in strengthening one's position with these gods was to win their favor by keeping one's conduct on a high moral plane; here the Taoists recommended such practical good deeds as feeding the poor, saving people from danger, and building roads and bridges. At the same time, sins had to be expiated by rituals of penitence. The second step was to aid with prayers the continual struggle of the body divinities against evil spirits and harmful breaths. For example, if one experienced a ringing in the ears, it was necessary at once to say a routine prayer. If the face subsequently became warm, then all was well; but if the face became cool, it was a dire sign that an evil spirit had succeeded in penetrating the body, and the adept had to rush to his home for urgent prayers to the highest divinities. The third method of retaining the body gods involved both mysticism and magic; this consisted of meditation and "interior vision" which allowed one to "see" the gods within his body. This procedure required a long apprenticeship, for the divinities had to be visualized precisely as they were described in scripture: the god of the hair, two inches high and dressed in gray; the god of the skin, one and a half inches high and dressed in yellow, etc.; and in each case he had to be seen in the correct pose, surrounded by the proper entourage. In this way, all the gods of the body were passed in review and, being visualized regularly, it was considered that they were not able to leave.

The deities of the outside world (macrocosm) also were wooed with ethical conduct and prayers, and communication was sought with them. Good deeds and supplications were directed especially towards the "Director of Destiny" (and his assistants) who controlled longevity, fixing at birth the life span of each individual and increasing or decreasing the allotment according to his religious merit. The attempts at communion, on the other hand, were aimed at the "Venerable Celestials," the angels of the Taoist system; these covered a wide variety of status, ranging from men who had recently become hsien or immortals all the way up to gods of high rank. Each adept endeavored to make contact with one of these guardian angels, for it was from them that one received the most valuable instructions on the techniques for prolongevity and immortality. The Venerable Celestials made their appearance in places of solitude, particularly on high mountains and in deep grottoes, and many a hopeful adept dissipated his life's savings as he wandered through remote areas of the countryside seeking contact with a divine protector.

One sought to establish relationships of this kind with deities higher and higher in the celestial hierarchy. Beyond this, there always remained the supreme goal of Taoism, direct communion with the tao itself; that is, the attainment of a state of mystic ecstasy in which one felt with certainty the presence of the tao within oneself; all ordinary worries and desires were annihilated; one's body had become identical with the subtle substance of the spirit; one was immortal.

CONCLUSION

Taoism's great achievement was to take prolongevitism from the realm of magic and carry it forward to a stage which is best termed proto-science. The Taoists did not originate the idea of prolongevity; what they did was to take the prolongevitist vagaries of folklore and form them into an organized body of concepts and hypotheses suitable for assimilation by science. Taoism was the first system of prolongevitism. Its service in that regard is made clearer by contrasting it with the paucity of comparable developments in the ancient and early-medieval West. In Greek science, the pre-Socratics played a pioneer role similar to that of the Taoists; but among the pre-Socratics the idea of prolongevity remained peripheral. Later Greek science was characterized by an overemphasis on the abstract and the logical; the utilitarian and meliorist aspects of science were underestimated. In Hellenic thought (Plato, Aristotle) there was too sharp a break with neolithic magic; the gap was too wide between matter and spirit, between man and the gods to allow the flourishing of that "natural magic" which was to be so fruitful in the early period of modern science.

Aside from its general intellectual significance, Taoist prolongevitism must be credited with specific ideas and practices which have enriched medicine and science in China and the West.[85] The Taoist sexual procedures, for example, passed into the regimen of Chinese medicine. The gymnastic techniques not only became an integral part of Chinese hygiene but, as we have seen, were transmitted to the West where they were incorporated into the Swedish system of medical gymnastics. The Taoist search for hsien foods and medicines added a great many substances to the Chinese pharmacopoeia. Perhaps the most productive of all was Taoist alchemy, especially if it can be shown that its store of chemical technology was passed to the West (via the Arabs). In general, historians of science are coming to recognize the high significance of the Chinese contribution to Western science and technology.[86] These Chinese achievements owed much to Taoism:

---

[85] The best source for these matters will be the complete Needham, SCC. The tentative table of contents for all volumes has been published in volume one.

[86] Needham points out that the three technical advances traditionally credited with the greatest impact in Western culture—printing, gunpowder, and the magnetic compass—all were derived from China; Needham, SCC 1: p. 19.

. . . many aspects of Chinese science, such as alchemy, pharmaceutical botany, zoology, and the physics of magnetism, are patently Taoist in inspiration.[87]

And it is well to recall that the chief motivation for these Taoist investigations of nature was the belief that it was desirable and possible to prolong the span of life.

Great as the achievements of Taoist prolongevitism were, its limitations were nearly as formidable. The Taoist attitude was too qualitative and subjective; any adept could supply his own data based on revelations from the Venerable Celestials, from "interior vision" or from other types of mystical insight. The result was a confusing proliferation of opposing schools and systems. Once accepted by a group of adepts, a teaching gained the status of scriptural authority; treatise after treatise was added to the canonical literature, and, lacking both the internal discipline of logic and the external discipline of ecclesiastical organization, Taoism became overly burdened with the spurious and the superstitious.

The shortcomings of Taoist prolongevitism demonstrate how serious a handicap it is for such a movement to be based on primitivism rather than on the idea of progress. To the Taoists the golden age was in the past. While this attitude may have been beneficial in allowing them to utilize traditional Chinese beliefs, at the same time it placed definite limitations on the acquisition of new knowledge. Their excessive veneration for the wisdom of the ancients saddled the Taoists with obsolete notions and severely checked the development of independent thinking. Even those who, like Ko Hung, were closest to the spirit of scientific inquiry could not escape this thralldom to the past. Ko Hung devoted many pages to attempts to refute the critics of prolongevitism, and his arguments relied heavily on legendary material of the antediluvian, fountain, and phoenix types. For him this folklore assumed scientific validity; he was unable to admit that even the sages might be ignorant as to the causes of old age. Lacking the idea of progress, he could not place his hopes in the future; he had to assert that prolongevity already had been achieved and was continuing to be achieved by a select few who, however, had chosen to veil their methods in obscurity. Such a rationale for prolongevitism could not resist the inroads of secrecy, ritualism, superstition, and charlatanism.

VI. THE ALCHEMISTS [1]

For that medicine which would remove all impurities and corruptions of a baser metal, so that it should become

---

silver and purest gold, is thought by scientists to be able to remove the corruptions of the human body to such an extent that it would prolong life for many ages.

Roger Bacon, *Opus majus* [2]

Alchemy is of prime significance for our study because it represents the first systematic prolongevitism to appear in Western civilization. We already have seen the strong position that apologism held in the West, and we also have drawn a contrast between the central role of prolongevitism in China and its meager status in Western thought. The prolongation of life remained a neglected theme in the West throughout antiquity and far into the Middle Ages until suddenly in the thirteenth century there appears a full-fledged prolongevitist alchemy. Then, not without surprise, one reads in the manifesto of Roger Bacon concerning the usefulness of experimental science:

Another example can be given in the field of medicine in regard to the prolongation of human life, for which the medical art has nothing to offer except the regimen of health. But a far longer extension of life is possible . . . the experimental art supplies the defect of medicine in this particular.[3]

Bacon was very apt in choosing to stress the dissimilarity between his "experimental science" of prolongevity and the traditional Galenic hygiene which attempted not to secure the utmost longevity possible but rather to guide each individual to his "natural span of life." [4] What Bacon offered was something radically new in the Western world: a methodical rationale for the possibility and desirability of prolonging life. And the "experimental science" on which he based his prolongevitism was, for the most part, alchemy.

This prolongevitist alchemy played a role of great importance in the history of ideas as well as in the history of science and medicine. For centuries it was one of the chief vehicles for the belief that through science man may gain extraordinary powers over nature, a line of thought which was to flower richly during the Enlightenment. In regard to science, it is well known that alchemy contributed the major part of the techniques and materials for the beginnings of modern chemistry;

---

[87] *Ibid.* 2: p. 493.

[1] The most satisfactory introduction to alchemy is F. Sherwood Taylor, *The Alchemists: Founders of Modern Chemistry,* Life of Science Library (New York, 1949); this work hereafter is referred to as "Taylor, *Alchemists.*" Also very useful is E. J. Holmyard, *Alchemy* (Harmondsworth, 1957); this work hereafter is referred to as "Holmyard, *Alchemy.*" Both studies lack annotation but are by recognized authorities. Still highly regarded for its thorough documentation, but somewhat out of

date in interpretation, is Edmund O. von Lippmann, *Entstehung und Ausbreitung der Alchemie* (3 v., Berlin, 1919–1931 and Weinheim, 1954). Superseded by Taylor and Holmyard, but worthy of mention, is Arthur John Hopkins, *Alchemy: Child of Greek Philosophy* (New York, 1934). An interesting account, but too unsystematic, is John Read, *Prelude to Chemistry: an Outline of Alchemy, its Literature and Relationships* (New York, 1937). Indispensable to students of the subject is *Ambix,* Jour. Society for Study of Alchemy and Early Chem., 1937 ff. A sound introduction to the history of chemistry, with good chapters on alchemy, is Henry M. Leicester, *The Historical Background of Chemistry* (New York and London, 1956). See also, Allen G. Debus, "The Significance of the History of Early Chemistry," *Jour. World History* 9 (1965): pp. 39–58.

[2] Roger Bacon, *Opus majus,* Robert Belle Burke, transl. (2 v., Philadelphia and London, 1928) 2: p. 627.

[3] Bacon, *op. cit.* (see fn 2), pp. 617–618.

[4] See earlier, chap. II, section on biology and medicine.

the prolongevitist school was involved particularly in the development of distillation techniques and the chemical uses of alcohol and the mineral acids. In medicine, the alchemy of long life led, through the work of John of Rupescissa and Paracelsus, to the rise of iatrochemistry, which, in turn, was the early antecedent for the biochemistry and chemotherapy of our own time.

An appreciation of alchemy is made difficult by the derision with which it customarily has been treated in general works of science and history. The origins of this prejudice are easily found. Even during the period of its greatest prestige, "the art" was raked by withering criticism from vested interests: the state and the propertied classes felt themselves threatened by the possibility that individual alchemists actually might succeed in transmuting base metals into gold; and the clergy and the medical profession were suspicious of the attempt by laymen to obtain a panacea for disease and an elixir of long life. The pretensions of alchemy were discredited further by the rise of modern chemistry, which, in its effort to cast off outmoded doctrines, did not hesitate to resort to sarcasm and ridicule. Finally, having been stripped of its ties with science, alchemy became the domain of religious mystics who elaborated from it a system of religious speculation known as Hermetic Philosophy. This mystical tendency was carried so far that some modern students of the subject concluded that the quest of the alchemist always had been symbolic and religious rather than material and scientific.[5] Because of these later developments, it requires an effort of the imagination to realize that, within the framework of ancient and medieval science, the hypotheses of the alchemists were quite valid and could be accepted by such learned men as al-Razi and Thomas Aquinas.[6]

Equally unfortunate is the tendency to identify alchemy with charlatanism. As F. Sherwood Taylor points out, a clear distinction usually can be drawn between genuine practices and pseudo-alchemy.[7] The bona fide adept was engaged in a difficult and time-consuming undertaking. First, there was the "gross work," the collection and purification of materials; then the "subtle work," the actual preparation of the elixir. All this required months and years of tedious effort fraught with the anxious knowledge that the least slip might nullify the entire procedure. Furthermore, the endeavors of the true alchemist required him to lead a sedentary existence, and the traditions of his calling swore him to prudence and secrecy regarding his research

and piety and morality in the conduct of his life. The demeanor and purposes of the false alchemist usually were in contrast with this: he professed to have a quick and easy method for preparing the elixir, he was an itinerant, and he was prepared, for a price, to demonstrate his skill in public.[8]

Even to the most unbiased scholar, however, the study of alchemy presents formidable obstacles. Only a small number of investigators have ventured into the wide ranges of alchemical literature, and it follows that many areas remain uncharted. Of the hundreds of treatises attributed to Jabir, for example, only a handful have been translated or even carefully examined. What is more, research in this field is handicapped by the ambiguity and obscurity of alchemical writings; from the very first, the adepts were obsessed with the need for secrecy. In the fourth century, Ko Hung warned that, ". . . disbelievers of the Way should not be given any information, for they would slander and spoil the elixir, and thus the Medicine will fail."[9] Therefore, ". . . secrecy is thrown over the efficacious recipes. . . . The substances referred to are commonplaces which nevertheless cannot be identified without knowledge of the code concerned."[10] The directions for preliminary processes often are straightforward enough, but as one approaches the heart of the matter, the preparation and use of the elixir, the clarity comes to an end, and one is left with vague, symbolic phrases, the explanation of which was transmitted only orally. This deliberate obscurity doubly confuses the modern reader who already finds the material refractory enough owing to its obsolete terminology and the archaic nature of its concepts and hypotheses.

Controversies in the interpretation of alchemy affect the definition itself.[11] In a narrow sense, alchemy may be defined as the art which sought to transmute ordinary metals into silver and gold, and which attempted to prepare a chemical medicine which would cure all diseases and greatly prolong life. Others would make a more sweeping generalization by stating that alchemy was chemistry before 1500. This larger definition has the advantage of reminding us that throughout antiquity and the Middle Ages, alchemy was the chief repository of chemical techniques and theories, and that it provided one of the main foundations for modern chemistry. It goes too far, however, in implying a comprehensiveness

[5] On the symbolic interpretation of alchemy, see I. Bernard Cohen, "Ethan Allen Hitchcock: Soldier, Humanitarian, Scholar—Discoverer of the 'True Subject' of the Hermetic Art," Proc. Amer. Antiquarian Society 61 (1951) : pp. 44–52, 64–79; Cohen discusses the ideas of Hitchcock, Atwood, Silberer and the famous C. G. Jung.

[6] Other savants, e.g., Avicenna and Albertus Magnus, were sceptical regarding applied alchemy but accepted the basic suppositions of alchemical theory.

[7] Taylor, Alchemists, pp. 105–107.

[8] A typical method of the alchemical quack was to place some gold beforehand inside a piece of charcoal, sealing it in place with black wax. After some mercury was added, the charcoal was ignited; the mercury was volatilized by the heat, the charcoal was burned away, and the melted gold was left in the receptacle.

[9] Ko Hung, Pao-p'u Tzu, chap. 4, Eugene Feifel, transl., Monumenta Serica (Peking) 9 (1944) : p. 10.

[10] Ibid., chap. 16, Lu-Ch'iang Wu and Tenney L. Davis, transl., Proc. Amer. Academy of Arts and Sciences 70 (1935) : pp. 262–263.

[11] For the definitions of alchemy, see Encyclopedia of Chemistry, George L. Clark, ed. (New York, 1957), pp. 28–29.

which alchemy did not have; Avicenna, for example, contributed to chemical knowledge but, at the same time, denied the possibility of alchemical transmutation in the laboratory. Two of the other components which went to make up modern chemical science were largely outside the realm of alchemy: the chemical crafts, such as dyeing and glassmaking, and the philosophical atomism which originated in ancient Greece and was revived in the seventeenth century by Boyle, Descartes, and Gassendi.

Our own inquiry will be different from previous ones, for most studies of the subject have been slanted towards chemistry *per se*.[12] We, however, are interested in alchemy as a school of prolongevitism and as a precursor of medical chemistry. Previous investigations, by and large, have sought an understanding of how the elixir was prepared, and why it was presumed to bring about the transmutation of metals. We pose a different question: why was it thought that the elixir could cause a significant extension of the length of life? With that purpose in mind, we shall examine the various stages of alchemical evolution: first, the Chinese, which arose in association with Taoism and was strongly prolongevitist; then, briefly, the Hellenist, in which prolongevitism was strikingly absent; then the Arabic, which often has been considered the carrier of prolongevity ideas from the East to the West; and finally the Latin, with its implications for iatrochemistry and the Enlightenment.

CHINESE ALCHEMY [13]

In all of world history, the first mention of alchemy occurs in China and is related to the prolonga-

tion of life. The passage is found in the work of Ssu-ma Ch'ien, the great historian who lived in the first century B.C.; in it, the alchemist Li Shao Chün advises the Han emperor Wu Ti (156–87 B.C.),

If you make sacrifice to the furnace, you will be able to transmute cinnabar into gold. When the gold shall have been produced, you may make of it utensils for eating and drinking. Through using them your life will be prolonged, so that you may see the blessed immortals of the island of P'eng Lai, which lies in the midst of the ocean. When you shall have seen them, and shall have made proper sacrifice to high heaven and broad earth—then you will never die.[14]

These sentences are so laden with historical significance that they deserve immediate elucidation. The "sacrifice to the furnace" is directed apparently to that "God of the Stove" who became one of the great Taoist divinities, Ssu-ming, the controller of longevity.[15] The idea that cinnabar may be transmuted to gold is extremely interesting because cinnabar is mercury sulphide, and it is a dominant hypothesis in all alchemy—Hellenist, Arabic, and Latin—that the principles of mercury and sulphur are the basis of metals. The notion that, by eating and drinking from golden vessels, one will lengthen one's life, is a recurrent theme in alchemy and medicine right down to modern times: it represents one method of getting gold into a potable and nontoxic form. Finally, the reference to the "immortals of the island of P'eng Lai" demonstrates the influence of folklore, for P'eng Lai is one of those Isles of the Eastern Sea which were discussed in chapter four as examples of the hyperborean theme.

Like the other Chinese prolongevity techniques, alchemy originated from a blending of primitive magic, traditional nature-philosophy and Taoist metaphysics.[16] It is a custom among neolithic peoples to deposit red pigment with the dead: in the West, this was red ochre

---

[12] I do not know of any previous study of the over-all relationship between alchemy and the prolongation of life. There is a French, medical-school thesis which attempts to sketch the relation between alchemy and medicine, but it is too elementary, unhistorical, and poorly documented; R. Allendy, *L'Alchimie et la médecine* (Paris, 1912). There are, however, some excellent studies of selected aspects of medical alchemy; e.g., Owsei Temkin, "Medicine and Graeco-Arabic Alchemy," *Bull. Hist. of Medicine* 29 (1955): pp. 134–153 and Robert P. Multhauf, "John of Rupescissa and the Origin of Medical Chemistry," *Isis* 45 (1954): pp. 359–367.

[13] The most authentic introduction to Chinese alchemy is provided by translations of works by Ko Hung and Wei Po-yang. For the alchemical section (20 chapters) of Ko Hung's *Pao-p'u Tzu*, see the translation of chapters 1, 2, 3, 4, and 11 by Eugene Feifel in *Monumenta Serica* (Peking) 6 (1941): pp. 113–211, 9 (1944): pp. 1–33, and 11 (1946): pp. 1–32; the translation of chapters 4 and 16 by Lu-ch'iang Wu and Tenney L. Davis in *Proc. Amer. Academy of Arts and Sciences* 70 (1935): pp. 221–284 and the translation of chapters 8 and 11 with summaries of all the other chapters by Ch'en Kuo-fu and Tenney L. Davis in *ibid.* 74 (1941): pp. 297–325. These works hereafter will be referred to as "Ko Hung, *Pao-p'u Tzu* (Feifel)," "(Wu)" and "(Ch'en)" respectively. See also, Wei Po-yang, *Ts'an T'ung Ch'i*, Lu-Ch'iang Wu and Tenney L. Davis, transl., *Isis* 18 (1932): pp. 210–289. Three useful secondary works are Masumi Chikashige, *Alchemy and Other Chemical Achievements of the Ancient Orient* (Tokyo, 1936); Obed S. Johnson, *A Study of Chinese Alchemy* (Shanghai,

1928); and William Jerome Wilson, "Alchemy in China," *Ciba Symposia* 2 (1940): pp. 593–624; the last of these includes a helpful bibliography. These works will be superseded to some extent on the completion of Joseph Needham, *Science and Civilization in China* (Cambridge, 1954 ff.). Nathan Sivin has begun an ambitious investigation in depth of Chinese alchemy; see his "Preliminary Studies in Chinese Alchemy: The *Tan Ching Yao Chueh*, Attributed to Sun Ssu-mo (581?–after 672)," unpublished doctoral thesis, Harvard U., 1965.

[14] Johnson, *op. cit.* (see fn. 13), pp. 76–77.

[15] Holmes Welch, "Syncretism in the Early Taoist Movement," *Papers on China* (duplicated for private distrib. by East Asia Program, Committee on Regional Studies, Harvard U.) 10 (1956): pp. 12–15.

[16] On the history of Chinese alchemy, in addition to the works of Chikashige, Johnson, and Wilson in footnote 13, see Tenney L. Davis and Lu-Ch'iang Wu, "Chinese Alchemy," *Scientific Monthly* 31 (1930): pp. 225–235; Homer H. Dubs, "The Beginnings of Alchemy," *Isis* 38 (1947): pp. 62–86; Arthur Waley, "Notes on Chinese Alchemy," *Bull. School of Oriental Studies* (London) 6 (1930): pp. 1–24; Welch, *op. cit.* (see fn. 15), pp. 10–19, 33–36 and also Welch, *The Parting of the Way: Lao Tzu and the Taoist Movement* (Boston, 1957), pp. 96–105, **126–132.**

(iron peroxide); in China, cinnabar was used. The general assumption is that this practice was founded on the magical notion associating the color red with blood and hence with life; from this, one can speculate, there arose the attempt to prepare a nontoxic form of cinnabar, so that it might be ingested for its life-preserving qualities.[17]

The general chemical rationale for the working up of cinnabar was provided by the theory of the five elements (earth, fire, water, metal, and wood) and the two principles (yin = passive, yang = active); this conceptual scheme is associated with the name of Tsou Yen, who probably wrote about 320 B.C.[18] Roughly contemporaneous with Tsou Yen were the Taoist classics, which, with their emphasis on the unity of nature, underscored the idea of transformation: that one substance might be changed into another, and that a man might be metamorphosed into an immortal or *hsien*.[19] These fundamental aspects of alchemy converged in the activities of Li Shao Chün, whose advice to Han Wu Ti may be dated as 133 B.C. After that there are occasional references to alchemical experiments at the imperial court until a notorious failure in 56 B.C. temporarily cast a pall over the subject; a cousin of the Emperor had received full financial backing but after four years was unable to produce an elixir of life.

The two outstanding names in Chinese alchemy are Wei Po-yang and Ko Hung.[20] Very little is known about the life of Wei Po-yang, but he is justifiably famous as the author of the first full treatise on the subject, the *Ts'an T'ung Ch'i* or "Relatedness` of the Trio," a title the meaning of which remains obscure; this influential work was written about A.D. 142. The personality of Ko Hung, on the other hand, has come down to us with unparalleled vivacity, for he produced the most complete autobiography in early Chinese literature. He lived approximately from A.D. 260 to 340, and his alchemical writings are included in the work which is known by his nickname of *Pao-p'u Tzu* or "Old Sober-Sides." Because of his early advocacy of medical chemistry, he has been termed the "Chinese Paracelsus," but in his career he reminds one of Francis Bacon. Like Bacon, Ko Hung was a high-ranking politician who became fascinated by science and its exciting possibilities for human control over nature and for the prolongation of life. And, like Bacon, he is renowned not as an original experimenter but as a compiler and popularizer with a very winning manner, as, for example, in this introduction to alchemy:

If we think of becoming acquainted with this science, we must be conscious of the fact that we leave a filthy cesspool and float on the great ocean; we are turning our back to the light of the fire-fly and face the sun and the

moon, we hear the peals of thunder and realize how mean the claps of the cloth-drum are.[21]

After Ko Hung, the data on Chinese alchemy becomes very scanty; there seems to have been little creativity. When the sources become more abundant after 900, it has become "internal" alchemy, a mystical and symbolic calling like the Hermetic Philosophy which developed in the West after 1500; that is, a discipline worked out by spiritual changes within the individual rather than by material operations in a laboratory.

Chinese alchemy was identified very closely with Taoism; in fact, nearly ten per cent of the titles in the Taoist scriptures, the *Tao Tsang,* refer to alchemy.[22] Even Ko Hung, who, in some respects, shows Confucian tendencies, began his alchemical text with a chapter glorifying the *tao* and praising the classical Taoist virtues of nonconformity and effortless action.[23] And his chemical techniques were performed in an aura of religious Taoism:

As in the case of the making of the nine medicines [elixirs], services of worship should be properly performed to *T'ai I, Hsuan Nü* and *Lao Tzu* in the making of the Yellow and the White [gold and silver]. There should be constant burning of the five incenses. When gold is successfully compounded, three pounds of it should first be thrown into deep water. . . .[24]

Among the prolongevity techniques of Taoism, alchemy had the greatest prestige; an adept who obtained the elixir became a *hsien* of the highest rank.[25] Ko Hung went further yet in declaring that, while ethical and physiological practices could prolong life, only alchemy actually could lead to immortality.[26]

The focal characteristic of Chinese alchemy is its nearly complete dedication to the goal of lengthening life. This is demonstrated in most detail in the writings of Ko Hung, who expended a great deal of effort in defence of prolongevitism. By and large, he assumed that everyone would agree on the *desirability* of longer life, although he did consider it necessary to loose a blast against the apologist tendencies within Taoism:

As to Wen-tzu, Chuang-tzu and Kuan-ling Yin Hsi . . . the final word is not there at all. Sometimes they equalize death and life, saying there is no difference. They consider life as hard labor and death as rest. . . . They are not worth bothering with.[27]

The great alchemist's most intensive concern was with the *possibility* of prolongevity, and to this question he devoted two chapters: "Discussion on Immortality" and "Answer to Common Belief." [28] Here he had to

[17] Waley, *op. cit.* (see fn. 16), pp. 18–19.
[18] On Tsou Yen, see Needham, *op. cit.* (see fn. 13) 2: pp. 232–244.
[19] See earlier, chap. IV, section on Taoist philosophy.
[20] For the writings of Wei Po-yang and Ko Hung, see fn. 13.

[21] Ko Hung, *Pao-p'u Tzu* (Feifel), chap. 4 in 9: p. 6.
[22] Davis and Wu, *op. cit.* (see fn. 16), p. 225.
[23] Ko Hung, *Pao-p'u Tzu* (Feifel), chap. 1 in 6: pp. 117–131.
[24] *Ibid.* (Wu), chap. 16, p. 268.
[25] Henri Maspero, *Le Taoisme* (Paris, 1950), pp. 96–97.
[26] Ko Hung, *Pao-p'u Tzu* (Ch'en), pp. 302, 322–323.
[27] *Ibid.* (Ch'en), chap. 8, p. 307.
[28] *Ibid.* (Feifel), chaps. 2 and 3 in 6: pp. 132–211.

meet the charge that, since death is an inevitable rule of nature, it is a waste of time to attempt to evade it. His first line of defense was to challenge the validity of this universal negative, i.e., that immortality is impossible; he criticized such a sweeping statement as arrogant and dogmatic in view of man's limited knowledge.

The space between heaven and earth is infinitely great; in it there are all kinds of strange things. Why then should there be a limit for them? . . . Our body is something that we ourselves possess, but nobody knows anything. about the reasons why our heart and feelings are such as they are. Life and destiny is attached to us, but nobody knows anything about the length of the days which we can attain.[29]

Ko Hung hammered away on the theme that natural phenomena are innumerable in variety and unpredictable in their interactions; astonishing transformations take place and marvelous powers are manifested. Is it not unreasonable to rule out arbitrarily the possibility of prolonging life?

We may perhaps be unable to make up our mind to believe that our life can be prolonged or that immortality can be obtained, but why are we reluctant to make a trial? If only a slight success should come out from this trial, gaining thereby only [sic] two or three centuries of life, would this not be still better than the early death of the masses?[30]

Switching to the attack, Ko Hung brought forth the traditional big guns of Taoist prolongevitism. First, there is the phoenix theme, the belief that there are plants and animals with prodigious life spans: the pine and cypress, the crane and tortoise, the snake, tiger, deer, hare, and toad.[31] Secondly, there is the antediluvian theme that in the distant past there were people who enjoyed remarkably long life. These sages of early times passed on to their disciples the secret of immortality, and there resulted a lineage of hsien, a fact supposedly verified by the records of history.

Shall we say that there are no immortals on earth? Well, but the records written down by wise men of former generations deal with nearly one thousand men. They all have their full names (in those biographies) with the complete story of their lives and deeds, so they are no untrue tales.[32]

There are hsien, asserted the alchemist, dwelling at all times on earth, but they prefer to conceal their true nature and pass unrecognized except by a few adepts.

The doctrine of transmutation, which is basic in all schools of alchemy, appeared in China at a very early date; in fact, it is there that we find the earliest statement of it. In the writings of Huai Nan Tzu in the second century B.C., there is expounded the evolution of minerals which occurs deep in the earth, the "baser" minerals developing by natural processes over many years into "nobler" minerals, culminating in silver and gold.

When the chhi of the central regions ascends to the Dusty Heavens, they give birth after 500 years to chüeh [realgar?]. This in its turn produces after 500 years yellow mercury, yellow mercury after 500 years produces yellow metal (gold). . . .[33]

It was this hypothesis of a natural metamorphosis of one mineral into another that inspired the alchemist's dream of the artificial transmutation of base metals into gold. The adept hoped, by gaining true insight into natural processes, to learn to speed up, in the laboratory, the evolution of the higher minerals.

The phenomenon of transformation was not limited to chemical events but was thought to occur also in living things and, most significant of all, among human beings. To Ko Hung, nature was far from having fixed species and categories; on the contrary, it was characterized by almost unlimited flux and variation.

If one says that all beings which have received the life-fluid should be immutable, then there are facts as, e.g., pheasants change into big oysters, sparrows into clams, earth insects get wings, water frogs flutter and fly, the Shui-li [a type of oyster] change into clams, the Hsing and Ling become maggots, moles become Ju [a kind of bird], putrid grasses become fire-flies, the iguanas become tigers, snakes become dragons; therefore, should these transformations, then, be all untrue?[34]

These "facts," drawn from Chinese tradition, are of a sort frequently found in ancient and medieval natural history in both East and West; the Arabic and Latin alchemists used the same sort of argument to support the idea of transmutation. Of course, remarkable metamorphoses do occur in nature, as, for example, the change of caterpillar to butterfly or tadpole to frog; also, as recently as the nineteenth century, rather naive notions still were current about the spontaneous generation of complex organisms from nonliving matter. What is unusual about Chinese alchemy is its sweeping extension of the doctrine of transformation to the human realm. Ko Hung cites such human changes as those of one sex into another, human beings into animals and vice versa and the dead restored to life.[35] This leads up to the concept of the hsien: just as common minerals can change to valuable ones, and lower animals can become higher forms, so, by Taoist practices, man can transform himself into a finer being, a hsien or immortal.

Next to transmutation, the key belief of Chinese al-

[29] Ibid., chap. 2, p. 145.
[30] Ibid., chap. 4 in 9: p. 8.
[31] Ibid., chap. 3 in 6: pp. 184–188. On the phoenix and antediluvian themes in Taoism, see earlier, chap. IV, section on magic and folklore.
[32] Ibid., p. 182. On the hsien literature, see earlier, chap. V, introduction.

[33] Needham, op. cit. (see fn. 13) 3: p. 640.
[34] Ko Hung, Pao-p'u Tzu (Feifel), chap. 2 in 6: pp. 142–143.
[35] Ibid., pp. 143–144. There are clinical counterparts to these types of human transmutation; the first and second, for example, might be based on observations of endocrine malfunction or psychotic changes. On resuscitation, cf. later, chap. VIII, section on Franklin.

chemy was vitalism, but it was a vitalism somewhat different from the modern sort. The Taoists accepted the vitalist teaching that there is in living things some unique property or principle which cannot be explained in mechanical terms alone. But they would not subscribe to the postulate of modern vitalism that there exists a sharp unbridgeable gap between the animate and inanimate domains. The point of view of Taoism is quite the opposite: all things in the world contain at least a small amount of the vital spirit or essence, and thus all things are, to some degree, "alive." Therefore, while the Taoists were vitalists, it was a vitalism that extended beyond biology to include the phenomena of physics and chemistry. This is not really surprising, since a strain of vitalism runs through all ancient and medieval chemistry: it was not finally expunged from inorganic chemistry till the overthrow of the phlogiston theory by Lavoisier near the end of the eighteenth century. To the Taoists, everything was made of "breath" of varying degrees of purity, and we already have seen how the Taoist concept of "breath" was associated with those of life and spirit and finally with the *tao* itself. It was this idea of an all-pervading "breath" that provided the lever for a vitalist interpretation of all natural events.

Vitalism and the unity of nature are the twin pillars which supported the rationale for the prolongevity techniques of Chinese alchemy.[36] As was noted in the previous chapter, the vital principle in the human organism was the *ching* or essence, a subtle and ethereal substance allied to "breath." The longevity of each individual was directly proportional to the quantity and quality of the vital principle in his body. In the words of the early alchemist Wei Po-yang,

The divine *ch'i* (air, spirit, ethereal essence). . . . Whoever retains it will prosper, and he who loses it will perish.[37]

Consequently, the purpose of the adept was to find or prepare substances rich in breath or essence and ingest them in order to increase his own life-force.

Although the alchemists never spelled out the exact mechanism by which the taking-in of alien essences would bring about the strengthening of one's own vital powers, it is not accurate, as some authors do, to dismiss the practice merely as a variety of sympathetic magic.[38] Taoist hypotheses had progressed beyond the stage of magic to that of proto-science. By and large, they explained the process of alchemical prolongevity as analogous to the digestion and assimilation of food: if ordinary foods can sustain the body's activities, how much more potent an effect must follow the eating of highly-vitalized substances.

Even the five cereals are capable of supporting human life. . . . How could it be otherwise than that the divine

medicine of first quality would be ten thousand times better for man than the five cereals![39]

Another analogy was that of the fuel which strengthens a flame:

Thus we derive strength for ourselves from an external substance just as lard feeds fire and so it cannot die out.[40]

This passage is especially interesting because it represents a Chinese counterpart to the oil-and-lamp analogy which appears in Western gerontology.[41]

These vitalized materials were the link between the physiological techniques and the alchemical techniques. Closely related to the dietary practices (discussed in the previous chapter), were the prolongevity foods; for example, eggs, peaches, broth of turtle, etc. More identified with alchemy, on the other hand, were the "*hsien* medicines"; to find them and prepare them required special skills. Ko Hung, for example, described a type of long-lived monkey that cannot be dispatched either by blows or by fire; only if one blocks its nostrils with a certain mineral can it be killed. If the brains of a number of these strange animals are mixed with herbs and ingested, one can lengthen one's life by five hundred years.[42] The great majority of *hsien* medicines were herbs or minerals, and they were extremely numerous; Ko Hung devoted an entire chapter to cataloguing them.[43]

In going through the list, one notices certain recurring features ascribed to such materials, and these suggest the sort of characteristics which the adept believed to signify a rich store of vital principle:

—shining, translucent, bright, starlike
—fluid, wet, self-moving, slippery, bloodlike
—shaped like man or animal (e.g., certain roots)
—strong taste, sweet, sharp, bitter
—red, scarlet, cinnabarlike, fire-colored.

This brings to mind the Western medieval doctrine of "signs," according to which God has given things outward characteristics which indicate, on the basis of intuitive analogy, their medicinal uses.[44] At the same time, it must be stated that the choice of a few of the substances enumerated by Ko Hung cannot be explained on such a basis, and one may assume that these were selected on empirical grounds.

The *hsien* medicines were classified in a hierarchical manner according to their efficacy in lengthening life:

---

[36] On the unity of nature, see earlier, chap. IV, section on Taoist philosophy.

[37] Wei Po-yang, *op. cit.* (see fn. 13), p. 238.

[38] E.g., Wilson, *op. cit.* (see fn. 13), p. 600.

[39] Ko Hung, *Pao-p'u Tzu* (Feifel), chap. 4 in 9: p. 5.

[40] *Idem.*

[41] On the lamp analogy, see earlier, chap. II, section on biology and medicine. The idea appears as late as M. F. X. Bichat, *Physiological Researches on Life and Death,* F. Gold, transl. (Boston, 1827), p. 168.

[42] Ko Hung, *Pao-p'u Tzu* (Feifel), chap. 11 in 11: pp. 13–14.

[43] *Ibid., passim.*

[44] A. C. Crombie, *Medieval and Early Modern Science* (2nd ed., 2 v., Garden City, N. Y., 1959) 1: p. 17. See also Pagel (see later, fn. 157), pp. 148–149.

at the bottom were the herbs, at the top, the most expensive minerals.[45] The naive reasoning behind some of these evaluations is revealed by Ko Hung's remarks on the limitations of herbs:

Drugs of vegetable origin will putrefy when placed in the ground. They will decompose when cooked, scorch when burnt. They cannot preserve themselves.[46]

The implication is that, if these substances cannot "preserve themselves," they must be lacking in the properties which bring about immortality.

It is evident that plants and trees can do no more than prolong life; they are not medicines capable of bestowing eternal life.[47]

Next above herbs are various minerals, such as copper sulphate and arsenic sulphide; then come the more precious minerals: pearls, mica and jade, in "liquified" form. After the type of criticism directed at herbs, it is interesting to note the same thought-process behind the endorsement of mica:

. . . if the five yün-mu [mica] are put right into a blazing fire, they will never be destroyed, and if buried under ground, they will never decay. For this reason they are able to bestow eternal life upon man.[48]

Then there were the numerous *chih* or "fungi," a category difficult to define; some really were fungi, but most were rare minerals with striking properties, such as luminescence, fluidity, or marked coloring. At the peak of prestige were silver and gold and, most desirable of all, cinnabar.

The supreme position of cinnabar in Chinese alchemy is quite remarkable, for in the alchemy of other cultures the red mineral plays only a minor role. A number of reasons can be advanced to explain the Taoist fascination with this substance. For one thing, the bloodlike color indicated the presence of life-giving qualities; as has been mentioned, neolithic peoples of China deposited the vermilion pigment with their dead. Not only is its appearance striking, but cinnabar also has highly unusual chemical reactions. Most "stones," when heated, turn to ashes, but mercuric sulphide becomes mercury:

$$HgS + O_2 \xrightarrow{\text{heat}} Hg + SO_2$$
$$\text{(red)}$$

Now mercury is an intriguing material, for it is the only one of the familiar metals which exists in liquid form at ordinary temperatures; the English name "quicksilver" suggests the vitalistic interpretation so readily given its behavior, for "quick" here connotes "living." What is more, when mercury is heated it

forms a red powder:

$$2\,Hg + O_2 \xrightarrow{\text{heat}} 2\,HgO$$
$$\text{(red)}$$

Modern chemistry recognizes this as mercuric oxide (HgO), but to the ancient alchemist it appeared that the original cinnabar had been restored. This interpretation seemed all the more justified because of a strange property of mercuric oxide; when heated it readily returns to mercury:[49]

$$2\,HgO \xrightarrow{\text{heat}} 2\,Hg + O_2$$
$$\text{(red)}$$

Thus, the alchemists observed a seemingly endless shuttling from a "living" (red) mineral to a "living" (fluid) metal:

$$2\,Hg + O_2 \underset{}{\overset{\text{heat}}{\rightleftharpoons}} 2\,HgO$$
$$\text{(fluid)} \qquad\qquad \text{(red)}$$

Here, they felt, was an immortal chemical which thrived on the same heating process that "killed" lesser materials.

Now the substance of cinnabar is such, that the more it is heated the more exquisite are its sublimations. . . . cinnabar, if burnt, will become mercury, and after having passed through a series of other sublimations it is again turned into cinnabar . . . and thus it enables man to enjoy longevity.[50]

It would be satisfying to be able to correlate the mercuric sulphide of Chinese alchemy with the mercury-sulphur theory of metals which was the core of Western alchemy; however, this can be done only in a general way. In the various Chinese schemes postulating the evolution of minerals, there was one in which cinnabar is the primal substance leading ultimately up to silver and gold, and this one system is close to the Western notion that metals are derived from mercury and sulphur.[51] But other Chinese evolutionary outlines began, not with cinnabar, but with different chemicals: rock salt, orpiment, realgar, lead. Similarly, while cinnabar was denominated an essential ingredient of elixirs for producing gold, it is disturbing to find some elixirs which do not contain it at all. The best way around the dilemma is to assume that the term "cinnabar" was used in the same ambivalent way that the terms "mercury" and "sulphur" were used in the West; i.e., just as "mercury" and "sulphur" denoted ideal principles or essences similar to, but not identical with,

[45] On this hierarchy, see Ko Hung, *Pao-p'u Tzu* (Feifel), chap. 11 in **11** and Chikashige, *op. cit.* (see fn. 13), pp. 28–38.
[46] Ko Hung, *Pao-p'u Tzu* (Feifel), chap. 4 in **9**: pp. 9–10.
[47] *Ibid.*, chap. 11 in **11**: p. 27.
[48] *Ibid.*, p. 16.

[49] This unique reaction enabled Priestley to discover oxygen in 1775; James B. Conant, ed., *The Overthrow of the Phlogiston Theory*, Harvard Case Histories in Experimental Science **2** (Cambridge, Mass., 1950), pp. 12–13, 38 ff. Perhaps by coincidence, Priestley happened to be at least a moderate prolongevitist; see later, chap. VIII, introduction.
[50] Ko Hung, *Pao-p'u Tzu* (Feifel), chap. 4 in **9**: pp. 5–6.
[51] On Chinese ideas about the evolution of minerals, see Needham, *op. cit.* (see fn. 13) **3**: pp. 636–641.

ordinary sulphur and mercury, so "cinnabar" could signify a vitalized substance related to, but finer than, ordinary cinnabar.

This idea of a super-cinnabar is borne out by the Chinese concept of the elixir: while ordinary cinnabar can prolong life, "sublime cinnabar" can work transmutations, changing base metals into gold or common men into *hsien*. This "sublime cinnabar" constituted a very active and powerful principle capable of refining whatever it comes in contact with; it is nearly identical with certain elixirs of Western alchemy which consisted of combinations of highly purified (or "sublime") "mercury" and "sulphur." Ko Hung described the preparation of nine kinds of "divine" cinnabar, any one of which could bring about the production of gold, cause immortality or resuscitate a person dead for less than three days.[52] "Flower of cinnabar," for example, was made from the following ingredients: realgar (arsenic disulphide), alum (aluminum and potassium sulphate), rock salt (sodium chloride), "lake" salt (ammonium chloride, urea, etc.), arsenic trioxide, oyster shells (calcium carbonate), "red stone fat," soapstone (magnesium silicate) and lead carbonate. The mixture was covered tightly with "six-one mud," a pastelike compound of six or seven minerals (its composition and preparation varied among different alchemists). This was heated for thirty-six days, and, if the resulting elixir were ingested for seven days, immortality would be attained. If, on the other hand, the elixir were added to mercury or lead, gold would be produced.

Modern chemists have suggested that some of these ancient procedures actually may have produced a small amount of gold, thereby leading the alchemists to infer that transmutation had occurred. The Japanese chemist Chikashige feels that the "red stone fat" in the flower-of-cinnabar recipe might have contained red gold-ore along with the usual iron oxides found in red clay.[53] This gold, when brought into contact with mercury, would form an amalgam with it (a process used in modern gold mining), and thus come to the attention of the alchemist. Lead is another substance which often contains traces of gold; when the elixir was added to lead and heated, the lead would oxidize and disappear as fumes, leaving behind a small quantity of gold.

Aside from real gold, the traditional alchemical formulas also formed alloys and compounds with the appearance of gold; one of these was "mosaic gold" (stannic sulphide), a useful compound of tin which was first produced in China.[54] The adepts were not at all discouraged because these forms of "artificial gold" differed in certain respects from natural gold, for they felt that

the metal created by alchemy must be superior to ordinary gold. An entire branch of the art, "the yellow and white," was devoted to the production of artificial gold and silver.[55]

The Taoists sought gold not as a form of wealth but as a means of prolongevity. Gold was the *hsien* metal; its relation to base metals was the same as that of the immortal to common men.

Gold is non-corruptible in its nature and is therefore the most valuable of things. The men of the art feeding on it attain longevity . . . the complexion becomes rejuvenated, hoary hair regains its blackness, and new teeth grow where fallen ones used to be. If an old man, he will once more become a youth; if an old woman, she will regain her maidenhood.[56]

The reason for the veneration of gold was its incredible (though correctly observed) resistance to chemical change; in the treatise of Wei Po-yang we read that,

When gold is placed in a hot fire it is not deprived of the brilliancy of its color. Since the days of the unfolding of the universe, the sun and the moon have not diminished in brightness nor has gold lost any weight.[57]

And in Ko Hung,

Yellow gold, if put in fire and melted a hundred times, will not be spoiled nor will it rot until the end of the world, though it is buried in the ground.[58]

Having obtained gold by one means or another, the adept labored to put it into potable form so that it might be ingested and assimilated by the body. One method, as we have seen, was simply to eat from vessels of gold, thereby taking in minute quantities of the precious metal. But the more frequent alchemical approach was to try to pre-digest the gold by long treatment with organic materials; the softened substance then was shaped into pills and swallowed.[59] Or the gold was placed in wine for extended periods and the ensuing liquor was drunk as "gold juice."[60]

HELLENISTIC ALCHEMY [61]

Alchemy arose in the West somewhat later than in China; the earliest traces of alchemical speculation ap-

---

[52] On recipes for the elixirs, see Ko Hung, *Pao-p'u Tzu* (Feifel), chap. 4 in **9**: pp. 10–33 and Chikashige, *op. cit.* (see fn. 13), pp. 39–54.

[53] Chikashige, *op. cit.* (see fn. 13), pp. 48–51.

[54] Ko Hung, *Pao-p'u Tzu* (Wu), introduction, p. 232 and chap. 16, pp. 264–265.

[55] *Ibid.*, chap. 16, pp. 256–268.

[56] Wei Po-yang, *op. cit.* (see fn. 13), pp. 240–241.

[57] *Ibid.*, p. 240.

[58] Ko Hung, *Pao-p'u Tzu* (Feifel), chap. 4 in **9**: p. 5.

[59] *Ibid.* (Wu), chap. 16, p. 267.

[60] *Ibid.* (Feifel), chap. 4 in **9**: p. 2.

[61] There are good introductions to Hellenistic alchemy in Taylor, *Alchemists*, pp. 18–67; Holmyard, *Alchemy*, pp. 13–30 and Leicester, *op. cit.* (see fn. 1), pp. 16–52. More detailed accounts are Lippmann, *op. cit.* (see fn. 1) 1, parts 1–3 and Marcellin Berthelot, *Les Origines de l'alchimie* (Paris, 1885) and *Introduction à l'étude de la chimie des anciens et du moyen-âge* (Paris, 1938). For primary sources, the standard compilation is Marcellin Berthelot, transl. and ed., *Collection des anciens alchimistes grecs* (3 v., Paris, 1888); see also F. Sherwood Taylor, transl., "The Alchemical Works of Stephanos of Alexandria," *Ambix* 1 (1937): pp. 116–139, 2 (1938): pp. 39–49.

peared about the first century, and the oldest extant writings are thought to have been composed about A.D. 300. The scene of this activity was the Egyptian metropolis of Alexandria, with its Hellenistic blending of Greek culture with those of other peoples of the Near East. Unfortunately, no vivid personality like Ko Hung can be identified with this school; the authors of whom we know are little more than names, and mostly pseudonyms at that, for they sought to gain for their writings the prestige of such revered figures as "Ìsis," "Hermes" or "Moses." Although their language was Greek, most of these writers seem to have been Egyptians and Jews. It was not long before translations began to be made into Syriac, a fortunate circumstance, for this Aramaic language was easily accessible to the Arabs when they conquered the Near East in the seventh century.[62]

The two chief components in the creation of Hellenistic alchemy were Egyptian craftsmanship and Greek philosophy. The artisans of Egypt long had been noted for their skill in contriving imitations of precious metals and gems. Their techniques took on a new significance when theories were formulated regarding the possibility of genuine transmutation. These theories adopted the chemical ideas of Aristotle, just as Chinese alchemy had borrowed from the nature-philosophy of Tsou Yen; instead of the traditional Chinese five elements, there were the Aristotelian four (air, earth, fire, and water). Also taken from Aristotle was the concept that metals evolve from two sorts of "exhalation" or vapor, one moist and the other dry; these became identified with "mercury" and "sulphur," the former being passive and feminine, while the latter was active and male, very much as in the Chinese yin and yang. The role which Taoism played in Chinese alchemy was taken in the West by Neoplatonism. As in the case of the Taoists, the Neoplatonist mystics indirectly performed a service for science by challenging a dogmatic rationalism and thereby opening the way for more intuitive interpretations of the data.[63] The Neoplatonists of the fourth century were exceptionally interested in marvels and magic, and during those years Hellenist alchemy received its characteristic form.

The Hellenistic alchemists differed most notably from the Chinese in having no concern with the prolongation of life. While the source materials have not yet been studied thoroughly, all the evidence available at present indicates their purpose was limited to the production of gold and silver (and occasionally other expensive substances) in order to gain wealth. There is no sign that they thought of gold as a potent medicine. This is rather strange, because in ancient Greece gold was regarded with the same sort of awe which it aroused in the Taoists; take, for example, the statement: "Gold is a child of Zeus; no moth nor worm can eat it away."[64] Yet when Pliny came to discuss "remedies derived from gold," he limited its use to comparatively minor external ailments, as warts and fistulas.[65] The Hellenistic alchemists did not depart from this prosaic view of the pharmaceutical uses of gold.

Helping to explain the absence of prolongevitism, there are two other features of Hellenistic alchemy: the paucity of links with medicine and the lack of the concept of an "elixir." Temkin, in his study of the relationship between medicine and alchemy, found no significant association until the time of the Arab Jabir.[66] Similarly, the "elixir" does not enter Western alchemy until the work of Jabir.[67] Unlike the Chinese, the Hellenistic alchemists did not have the idea of a unique substance of enormous power capable of perfecting all things; their approach was the more painstaking one of instilling the properties of gold into matter that had been "killed," or brought back to its primary state. The closest they came to an elixir was in the "divine water," a term applied to various solutions useful in transmutation. In one highly unusual passage this "divine water" takes on semi-medical attributes: it heals every disease, makes the blind see and the deaf hear, resuscitates the dead and makes the living die.[68] However, this is an isolated example, and, furthermore, one cannot consider as an elixir of life a substance which "makes the living die." Also the general import of the work indicates that the passage is meant in a symbolic or metaphorical sense.

ARABIC ALCHEMY: THE MISSING LINK?[69]

Surprising as it may seem, it is difficult to find any explicit prolongevitism in Arabic alchemy. This is con-

[62] A collection of the Syriac material is Marcellin Berthelot, *Histoire des sciences: la chimie au moyen âge* 2: *L'Alchimie syriaque* (Paris, 1893).

[63] Adolph Harnack and John Malcolm Mitchell, "Neoplatonism," *Encyclopaedia Britannica* (11th ed., Cambridge, 1910–1911).

[64] C. R. Haines, transl., *Sappho: the Poems and Fragments* (London and New York, 1926), p. 126; the words in this fragment sometimes are attributed to Sappho, sometimes to Pindar.

[65] Pliny, *Natural History*, book 33, chap. 25 in John Bostock and H. T. Riley, transl. (6 v., London, 1855 ff.) 6: pp. 106–107.

[66] Temkin, *op. cit.* (see fn. 12).

[67] Taylor, *Alchemists*, p. 66.

[68] Temkin, *op. cit.* (see fn. 12), p. 145.

[69] The most authoritative introduction to Arabic alchemy (unfortunately not annotated) is Holmyard, *Alchemy*, pp. 58–101; see also Taylor, *Alchemists*, pp. 76–94. Essential in this field, and one of the finest studies ever made in the history of ideas, is Paul Kraus, *Jabir ibn Hayyan: contribution à l'histoire des idées scientifiques dans l'Islam*, Mémoires présentés à l'Institut d'Égypte 44 (Cairo, 1943), 1: *Le Corpus des écrits Jabiriens*; 2: *Jabir et la science grecque*; this work hereafter is referred to as "Kraus, *Jabir*." Two other outstanding students of Arabic alchemy are Julius Ruska and Henry Ernest Stapleton. Ruska's best known works are *Tabula Smaragdina: ein Beitrag zur Geschichte der hermetischen Literatur* (Heidelberg, 1926) and *Turba philosophorum: ein Beitrag zur Geschichte der Alchemie*, Quellen und Studien zur Geschichte der Naturwissenschaften und der Medizin 1 (Berlin, 1931). Stapleton's major articles appeared in *Memoirs Asiatic Society of Bengal* (Calcutta); they are: "Sal Am-

trary to what one would expect, for certain writers on alchemy mention the elixir of life as a goal of the Arabic alchemists; Taylor, for example, states this clearly:

It is certainly notable that the idea of the elixir as a medicine prolonging life was present to the Arabs and not to their Greek-speaking predecessors.[70]

Others imply the same thing but put the matter more indirectly, as Holmyard:

. . . Chinese alchemy was very predominantly intent upon. preparing a medicine that should ensure immortality: but this alchemical trend does not appear in Near Eastern alchemy until the days of Islam. . . .[71]

These assertions seem to be based largely on the following syllogism: There was no prolongevitism in Hellenistic alchemy; prolongevitism was an outstanding feature of both Chinese and Latin alchemy; therefore, prolongevitism must have been carried by Arabic alchemy from China to the West.[72]

The actual foundations of Arabic alchemy were provided by Hellenistic alchemy which, by the time of the Arab conquests in the seventh and eighth centuries, had spread from Alexandria to Syria and Iraq. Traditionally, the first important alchemic adept was Khalid ibn Yazid, a prince of the Damascus caliphate in the late seventh century, but the two really creative figures in Arabic alchemy were Jabir and al-Razi.[73] The career of Jabir is obscured by the legendary material which later became associated with his name; according to the most likely account, he was an Arab born in Mesopotamia and practiced the art at the court of the renowned caliph Harun al-Rashid in Baghdad during the late eighth century. His writings were the nucleus for a vast accumulation of treatises; all claim his authorship, but most show the imprint of ideas from the ninth and tenth centuries.

The Jabirian *corpus* is noted for its elaborate theories of the elixir, which are set forth in highly imaginative terms.[74] In contrast to the Jabirian works are those of al-Razi, which are of a sober and methodical character; where Jabir is identified with brilliant, if speculative, theorizing, al-Razi is known for his practical handbooks of alchemical materials and techniques.[75] This is the same al-Razi, the Persian of the ninth century, whose medical writings won him a foremost position among Arabic physicians. The other great medical authority of the Middle Ages, the early eleventh-century Persian, Avicenna, was the spokesman for those opposed to experimental alchemy; while he accepted the natural evolution of minerals within the earth, Avicenna doubted the possibility. of transmutation in the laboratory.[76] In addition to Jabir and al-Razi there were many lesser alchemists, a notable example being Maslama al-Majriti, who worked in Spain during the tenth century and performed some of the earliest quantitative studies (weight changes) in chemistry.[77] From Spain, and perhaps also Sicily, during the twelfth century, alchemy was transplanted to the rest of Europe as part of the great series of translations which introduced Arabic science and philosophy to the Latin West.

It is easy to see why Arabic culture has come to be thought of as the transmitter of Chinese alchemy to the West. At its height, the Arab empire reached to the borders of inland China, and, at the same time, Arab ships were trading with the ports of southern China. Moreover, certain features of Arabic alchemy suggest Chinese influence. The Arabic idea of the elixir, for example, seems more in keeping with Chinese concepts than with anything in Hellenistic alchemy. Also, the Arabic use of organic materials for the preparation of the elixir cannot be traced to Greek sources but might have come from China, where some of Ko Hung's recipes used similar substances. The Arabs placed a high value on sal ammoniac (ammonium chloride and carbonate) derived from the distillation of human hair, and Stapleton believes the Arabic term for the sharply saline chemical, *nushadur*, was derived from the Chinese *nau-sha*.[78] The name of another familiar material of Arabic alchemy is even more suggestive of Far Eastern origin: *kharsini* or "Chinese iron." [79] It is on the basis of this sort of evidence that Dubs has stated:

Arabic alchemy is so similar to prior Chinese ideas that its derivation from China is certain.[80]

moniac: a Study in Primitive Chemistry," 1 (1905): pp. 25–41; with R. F. Azo, "Alchemical Equipment in the Eleventh Century, A.D.," 1 (1905): pp. 47–71; with R. F. Azo, "An Alchemical Compilation of the 13th Century, A.D.," 3 (1910): pp. 57–94; with R. F. Azo and M. Hidayat Husain, "Chemistry in Iraq and Persia in the 10th Century A.D.," 8 (1927): pp. 317–417; these works hereafter will be referred to as "Stapleton: *Bengal* (1905a), (1905b), (1910) and (1927)" respectively. The classical collection of sources is Marcellin Berthelot, *op. cit.* (see fn. 62), 3: *L'Alchimie arabe*; this work hereafter is referred to as "Berthelot, *Arabe.*" For other important translations, see later, fn. 82 and 83.

[70] Taylor, *Alchemists*, p. 71.
[71] Holmyard, *Alchemy*, p. 39.
[72] This argument appears repeatedly with Wilson, *op. cit.* (see fn. 13), p. 619; Dubs, *op. cit.* (see fn. 16), pp. 84–85; F. Sherwood Taylor, "The Origins of Greek Alchemy," *Ambix* 1 (1937): pp. 32–33, and Tenney L. Davis, "The Problem of the Origins of Alchemy," *Scientific Monthly* 43 (1936): pp. 556–558.
[73] The best available history of Arabic alchemy is Holmyard, *Alchemy*, pp. 58–101.

[74] For a meticulous descriptive catalogue of the Jabirian *corpus*, see Kraus, *Jabir* 1.
[75] On al-Razi's alchemical career, see .Stapleton, *Bengal* (1927) and Julius Ruska, "Die Alchemie ar-Razi's," *Der Islam* 22 (1935): pp. 281–319.
[76] For Avicenna's ideas on chemistry, see E. J. Holmyard and D. C. Mandeville, transl., *Avicennae De congelatione et conglutinatione lapidum* (Paris, 1927).
[77] E. J. Holmyard, "Maslama al-Majriti and the *Rutbatu'l-Hakim*," *Isis* 6 (1924): pp. 293–305.
[78] Stapleton, *Bengal* (1905a).
[79] On *kharsini*, see *ibid.* (1927), pp. 405–407; also mentioned are "Chinese copper" and a "Chinese mirror," pp. 387–408.
[80] Dubs, *op. cit.* (see fn. 16), p. 84.

Nevertheless, a statement like that of Dubs rests on shaky foundations, for the evidence linking Arabic alchemy with the Chinese is indirect. In deriving their lineage, the Arabic alchemists themselves emphasized their ties with the Hellenistic tradition. Only once have I seen China mentioned in this connection: Ibn al-Nadim in the tenth century gave it as his opinion that the homeland of alchemy was Egypt, but added that there were others who traced the art to Persia, Greece, India, "or even China." [81]

Besides the testimony of the alchemists themselves, who, with this minor exception, associated themselves with the Greeks, there are other serious discrepancies between Arabic and Chinese alchemy. The concept of the *hsien,* for example, does not appear in Arabic alchemy. Furthermore, cinnabar, which had a cardinal place in China, receives only the most casual mention by the Arabs. As to organic materials, while Ko Hung used them, he considered them much less valuable than mineral substances; this is quite the opposite of Jabir, who esteemed organic ingredients more than the inorganic.

The most striking hiatus in the chain of evidence linking Chinese and Islamic alchemy is the paucity of references to prolongevity in the Arabic literature. In China, prolongevitism was the heart and soul of alchemy, but the Arabs virtually ignore the subject. It is revealing that those statements of Taylor, Dubs, Holmyard and Davis which speak of a continuity of prolongevitism from China to the Arabs are not backed up with citations from primary sources. Moreover, one fails to find explicit concern with the lengthening of life in the sources available in translation: the *Book of Ostanes* (extracts), the *Book of al-Habib,* "Manuscript 1074" (extract), the *Book of Crates* (about A.D. 800), the *Book of the Silvery Water and Starry Earth* (extracts) by Ibn Umail (tenth century), *The Sage's Step* (synopsis) by al-Majriti (late tenth century), the "Letter on Alchemy" by Ibn Bishrun (about A.D. 1000), selections from the anonymous "Essence of the Art" (A.D. 1034), the *Book of Knowledge Acquired Concerning the Cultivation of Gold* by al-Iraqi (thirteenth century) and the volume of miscellaneous treatises (extracts) from the library at Rampur.[82] In addition to these works by lesser figures, one must add nine important treatises by Jabir and three works by al-Razi.[83]

Especially noteworthy are the passages which reasonably could be expected to touch on prolongevity, but which, nonetheless, avoid the topic. For example, the definitions center entirely on transmutation: Ibn al-Nadim defined alchemists simply as "those who make gold and silver from other metals"; al-Razi defined the elixir as the "medicine" which converts metals to silver and gold; and Ibn Khaldun gave this formal definition of alchemy:

This is a science which studies the substance [elixir] through which the generation of gold and silver may be artificially accomplished, and comments on the operation leading to it.[84]

Similarly, in the polemical literature, one finds prolongevity neither as a matter for boasting by the alchemists nor as an object of ridicule by their enemies. Ibn Khaldun's critique of alchemy culminated in the objection that transmutation is against the will of God; probably, had he known of any prolongevitism among the alchemists, he would have included it in his charge of impiety, for he had earlier stated that the life of a Muslim is set at sixty or seventy years.[85] In the Latin Geber, which derives from Arabic sources, the alchemist faced the question that, if it takes nature a thousand years to perfect metals, how can an alchemist accomplish this, if his length of life cannot exceed a hundred years? Far from challenging the statement about the fixity of the life span, the alchemist accepted it at once and proceeded to argue the matter on other grounds.[86] There also appear in the Arabic alchemical literature extensive discussions of the extraordinary properties of things; all sorts of marvels are described, even the artificial creation of animals and men, but there seems to be nothing about prolongevity.[87]

Obviously, the prolongation of life was not a main theme of Arabic alchemy as it had been in Chinese; nevertheless, one cannot rule out conclusively the possibility that there may have been a current of prolongevitism among the Islamic adepts. The primary sources have not yet been studied well enough to justify a sweeping statement: for example, we know at least a thousand titles of treatises ascribed to Jabir; of these, several

---

[81] Berthelot, *Arabe,* p. 40. *Cf.* al-Iraqi and al-Majriti who cited numerous authorities, nearly all of them obviously either Hellenistic or Arabic; Abu'l-Qasim al-Iraqi, *Book of Knowledge Acquired Concerning the Cultivation of Gold,* E. J. Holmyard, transl., Librairie orientaliste (Paris, 1923) and Holmyard, *op. cit.* (see fn. 77), pp. 299–300, 302.

[82] The first four treatises are in Berthelot, *Arabe,* pp. 44–125. For Ibn Umail, see M. Turab 'Ali, H. E. Stapleton and M. Hidayat Husain, "Three Arabic Treatises on Alchemy by Muhammad Bin Umail," *Memoirs Asiatic Society of Bengal* (Calcutta) 12 (1933): pp. 1–213. For al-Majriti, Holmyard, *op. cit.* (see fn. 77). The letter of Ibn Bishrun is in Ibn Khaldun, *The Muqaddimah: an Introduction to History,* Franz Rosenthal, transl., Bollingen Series 43 (3v., New York, 1958) 3: pp. 230–245. The "Essence of the Art" is in Stapleton,

[Bengal] *(1905b)*; for al-Iraqi, see earlier, fn. 81; the Rampur treatises are discussed in Stapleton, *Bengal* (1910).

[83] The Jabirian treatises are in Berthelot, *Arabe,* pp. 126 ff. For the works by al-Razi, see Stapleton, *Bengal* (1910) and (1927); and Julius Ruska, *Al-Razi's Buch Geheimnis der Geheimnisse,* Quellen und Studien zur Geschichte der Naturwissenschaften und der Medizin 6 (Berlin, 1937).

[84] For these definitions, see Berthelot, *Arabe,* p. 26; Stapleton, *Bengal* (1927), p. 355; and Ibn Khaldun, *op. cit.* (see fn. 82) 3: p. 227.

[85] Ibn Khaldun, *op. cit.* (see fn. 82) 3: pp. 276–280; 1: p. 343.

[86] Geber, *Works,* Richard Russell, transl. and E. J. Holmyard, ed. (London and New York, 1928), pp. 34, 41.

[87] On marvelous properties of things, see Berthelot, *Arabe,* pp. 150–155 and Kraus, *Jabir* 1: pp. 141–154.

hundred manuscripts are extant, but not more than sixty-three have been published, even in part, and only ten of these in translation.[88] In the case of al-Razi, we have the names of twenty-six books, only four of which are extant.[89] These facts, of themselves, however, do not generate bounding hopes of finding an extensive literature of prolongevitism in Arabic alchemy, for neither Kraus' elaborate catalogue of the Jabirian *corpus* nor Ruska's careful study of the al-Razi material suggests anything of the sort. Nevertheless, it gives one pause to consider that Jabir was supposed to have written five hundred works on medicine, and of these we have only one manuscript and ten titles.[90] At any time, the discovery of a new manuscript, or the further study of an existing one, may upset present ideas about Arabic alchemy.

Meanwhile, how are we to account for the fact that the Latin alchemists traced their prolongevity ideas to the Arabs? The most likely explanation is that the Latin translators misread or misinterpreted the Arabic sources. While there seems to be no explicit prolongevitism in the Arabic literature, there are several facets of Arabic alchemy which could be adapted to support prolongevitism. Four of these features deserve special attention: (1) the strong ties between Arabic alchemy and medicine, (2) the concept of the elixir, (3) the use of the elixir to cure disease, and (4) the attitude towards human control over the natural world. The situation is similar to that which we dealt with in chapter IV, in seeking the origins of Taoist prolongevity. Classical Taoism was not clearly prolongevitist, but it included certain tenets which could be turned to account by prolongevitist commentators. In the same way, there seems little or no outspoken prolongevitism in Arabic alchemy, but the four characteristics just mentioned could have been sufficient to initiate a school of Latin alchemy seeking increased longevity.

1. The association between Arabic alchemy and medicine was a very close one. Both of the most influential writers, Jabir and al-Razi, were physicians.[91] Following in their footsteps, the other adepts made frequent use of medical analogies, speaking of the elixir as a "medicine" which overcomes the "diseases" of the base metals. Jabir even had attempted to create a complete theory of transmutation based on the physiology of Galen. According to Galen, there were in the body four humors (blood, phlegm, black bile, and yellow bile), and these in turn represented combinations of the four qualities: heat, cold, dryness, and wetness.[92] The balance of the

four qualities (or four humors) determined health and disease: if they were in balance, the individual enjoyed good health; if the balance became seriously disturbed, illness ensued; if the imbalance were severe enough, death resulted, i.e., the soul left the body. In a similar way, minor shifts in equilibrium determined one's temperament (sanguine, phlegmatic, etc.) or reflected one's age (youth was hot and moist, old age was cold and dry). What Jabir did was to project this Galenic system onto the problems of inorganic chemistry; he sought to identify the characteristic make-up or balance of the qualities in each metal and chemical substance.[93] By establishing an exact quantitative measurement of the qualities, he hoped to be able to alter the balance in one direction or another to produce any material desired.

2. Jabir's elixir was a mixture of "pure" qualities, in such proportion as to redress the balance in base metals and "cure" them, i.e., transmute them to gold.[94] The true Jabirian alchemist devoted himself to involved procedures designed to isolate the pure qualities for the elixir. Water, for example, according to Jabir, consisted of cold plus wetness plus "substance"; after many distillations, the wetness was removed, and there remained a white powder which was considered pure cold (and "substance"). The discussions of the theory of balance in physiological terms opened the way for passages which seem to verge on prolongevitism; thus, Jabir stated:

If you could take a man, dissect him in such a way as to balance his natures [qualities] and then restore him to life, he would no longer be subject to death. . . . This equilibrium once obtained, they will no longer be subject to change, alteration or modification and neither they nor their children ever will perish.[95]

And Ibn Bishrun wrote:

Man suffers from the disharmony of his component elements. If his elements were in complete harmony and [thus] not affected by accidents and (inner) contradictions, the soul would not be able to leave his body. Man would then live eternally.[96]

These analogies to physiology appear to be meant only as illustrations of what took place when base metals were balanced by the elixir; the result was gold, the immortal unchanging metal. There is no indication that the taking of the elixir would lead to human immortality; such an interpretation seems to have been blocked by religious considerations, as is revealed in this statement by Jabir:

It is thus that God has created man; if He had wanted him to be immortal, He would have placed in his being concordant elements rather than divergent ones. . . . As God does not want any being to subsist forever, besides

[88] Kraus, *Jabir* 1: p. 175.
[89] Ruska, *op. cit.* (see fn. 75), pp. 283–286.
[90] Kraus, *Jabir* 1: p. 155.
[91] On Jabir's medical works, see Kraus, *Jabir* 1: pp. 155–160. On the medical career of al-Razi, see Arturo Castiglioni, *A History of Medicine*, E. B. Krumbhaar, transl. (2nd ed., New York, 1947), pp. 267–270.
[92] On Galenic physiology and pathology, see earlier, chap. II, section on biology and medicine.

[93] On Jabir's theory of balance, see Kraus, *Jabir* 2: pp. 187–236 and Berthelot, *Arabe*, pp. 139–162.
[94] On the Jabirian elixir, see Kraus, *Jabir* 2: pp. 1–18.
[95] Berthelot, *Arabe*, p. 148.
[96] Ibn Khaldun, *op. cit.* (see fn. 82) 3: p. 232.

Himself, He has afflicted man with this diversity of the four natures which leads to death and the separation of the soul from the body.[97]

How different this is from Ko Hung and the Chinese alchemists! Nevertheless, it is possible to see how less literate, or perhaps less scrupulous, Latin scholars might reverse the field in regard to the balance theory and envision the application of the elixir for the prolongation of life.

While Jabir, with his concept of balance, attempted to fashion a more fundamental and precise theory of the elixir, he was not able to dispense entirely with the old vitalist and pantheist outlook. In the Jabirian *corpus,* and more insistently in the works of others, there appears the same sort of naive speculation which characterized Taoist alchemy. The whole world is permeated with a cosmic spirit or breath[98]; this spirit (or breath) is found also in minerals where it plays the directing role in the evolution of the higher metals; the aim of the alchemist is to concentrate this vital spirit in an elixir or "philosopher's stone" with which he can accelerate the transmutation of metals. Thus, we read in Ibn Bishrun that,

Minerals contain substances, spirits and breaths which, when they are mixed and treated, produce something that may exercise an influence.[99]

By collecting these breaths in an elixir, one may perform "the operation," i.e, transmutation, as we read in the Jabirian *corpus,*

. . . the operation is practiced via concentrated things which contain a great quantity of spiritual force, subtle and light.[100]

The process of transmutation was compared with organic phenomena, especially the leavening of a large amount of dough by a bit of yeast.[101] In line with this vitalist interpretation, some alchemists, in the preparation of the elixir, preferred to use animal products: hair, blood, bile, etc.[102] In many of these discussions, minerals were spoken of as being alive and possessing bodies which were given eternal health by medicines consisting of concentrated spirits. It readily can be envisioned how passages of that nature, when read by Latin alchemists with only a limited command of Arabic, might have kindled hopes of prolongevity.

3. The actual use of the elixir to cure human disease is described in several remarkable case histories in the Jabirian *Large Book of Properties.* In one of these, Jabir told how he was called by the vizier to minister to a favorite slave-girl who seemed mortally ill; all the usual methods of treatment had been unavailing.

I saw her almost dead, her strength very much depleted. But I had a little of the elixir with me and of this I made her drink the amount of 2 grains in 3 oz. of pure oxymel. By God and by my Master, I had to cover my face before the maiden, for in less than half an hour her perfection was restored even to a higher degree than she had formerly possessed.[103]

Another case involved a slave of Jabir who had unwittingly taken a large dose of arsenic. None of the ordinary antidotes seemed able to counteract the poison.

Then I had him drink a grain (of this elixir) with honey and water. The instant it entered his body, he vomited all the arsenic and was restored to health.[104]

A third story concerned a man who had been bitten by a viper; subsequently his right side became swollen and ominously discolored green and blue.

I immediately had him drink 2 grains (of this elixir) dissolved simply in cold water, for I believed him to be on the point of death. By God, the green and blue colors disappeared and were replaced by the natural color of the body. Then the swelling decreased and disappeared. Having recovered his speech, he got up and returned home, entirely cured.[105]

Jabir asserted that with the elixir he had saved the lives of more than a thousand persons.[106]

4. Along with the medical uses of alchemy, the Arabic adepts made another significant contribution to the Latin world: the idea that science was the means for attaining human mastery over the forces of nature. Alchemy sought to capture for man's use the key to enormous powers over nature, the elixir with its marvelous cure of diseases and its transmutation of tens of thousands of times its own weight of ordinary metal into gold. All this was to be accomplished, not by some magic formula, but by arduous and systematic laboratory procedures based on credible theories of chemistry and biology. Jabir held unusually high hopes for his alchemical science; like Descartes, he felt that his scheme of thought had achieved the certainty of mathematics.[107] To Jabir, every natural phenomenon was simply the result of a concourse of forces which could be analyzed and controlled; not only could one produce artificial minerals, but one might hope even to create plants and animals.

The methods for doing this were not spelled out in detail, but the general principles were enunciated in accordance with the theory of the balance. To create a bird, for example, one must produce some sort of combination of egg white with airy and humid matter.[108]

[97] Berthelot, *Arabe,* p. 173.
[98] On cosmic breath, see the commentary on the "Emerald Table" in Holmyard, *Alchemy,* pp. 95–96.
[99] Ibn Khaldun, *op. cit.* (see fn. 82) 3: p. 239.
[100] Berthelot, *Arabe,* p. 177.
[101] E.g., *idem* and Ibn Khaldun, *op. cit.* (see fn. 82) 3: p. 268.
[102] Ibn Khaldun, *ibid.* 3: pp. 237–239 and Stapleton, *Bengal* (1905a), p. 28.

[103] Temkin, *op. cit.* (see fn. 12), p. 145.
[104] My translation from Kraus, *Jabir* 1: p. xxxix, fn. 6.
[105] *Idem.*
[106] Temkin, *op. cit.* (see fn. 12), p. 144.
[107] Jabirian optimism is analyzed in Kraus' brilliant section on artificial generation; Kraus, *Jabir* 2: pp. 97–135.
[108] *Ibid.,* p. 109.

For a creature of lesser intelligence, the balance would have to be shifted towards earth and water, for greater intelligence, towards air and fire.[109] What was original here was not so much the hypothesis of the balance, but the assertion that one might apply the hypothesis to alter, and even improve upon, nature. In considering such projects, Arabic alchemy veered perceptibly from primitivism towards the idea of progress.[110]

Perpetual progress in (this art) takes place because successive discoveries of men manifest themselves. . . . Thus someone is the initiator (of a science) and his successor, although less wise than he, catches up and, in a second attempt, surpasses him. . . .[111]

These Arabic speculations on the possibilities for the conquest of nature found an effective popularizer in Roger Bacon.

LATIN ALCHEMY [112]

Along with the other branches of Arabic science and philosophy, alchemy was introduced into Western Europe via Spain and Sicily during the twelfth century. The first recorded translation of an alchemical treatise was made in 1144 by Robert of Chester; another work was translated by the famous Adelard of Bath, and several more were done by the dean of translators, Gerard of Cremona. The imprint of Arabic remains in such terms as "alchemy," "alkali" and "naphtha," and the chief handbook of medieval Latin alchemy was ascribed to "Geber." Present-day scholars have not been able to trace the work of the Latin Geber to the Jabirian *corpus* or, indeed, to any other Arabic writing, but there is no doubt that it is based largely on Arabic ideas.[113]

At any rate, by the thirteenth century, alchemy was being widely discussed and practiced in Europe. The fundamental premises of the art were quite in keeping with scholastic natural history, for it generally was accepted that there was a natural evolution of minerals within the earth. It is not certain whether Albertus Magnus believed this transformation to be possible in the laboratory, but his successor Thomas Aquinas did accept the possibility of alchemical transmutation.[114] The great figure in the popularization of alchemy in this

initial period was Roger Bacon, who stressed its usefulness for the prolongation of life.

The two most revered names in fourteenth-century alchemy were Arnald of Villanova and Ramon Lull; both were natives of Catalonia, had a reading knowledge of Arabic, and were associated with semi-heretical religious movements.[115] Arnald, a preeminently successful physician, actually wrote only a few of the many alchemical works attributed to him; however, the lustre of his reputation helped to establish ties between alchemy and medicine. Ramon Lull, a mystical philosopher who died a martyr's death as a missionary among the Muslims of North Africa, is known to have been opposed to the hypothesis of transmutation. Nevertheless, a large number of writings claimed his authorship, and this Lullian *corpus* was extremely significant, as will be seen, because it embodied a new type of alchemy directed towards isolating the "quintessence." Other outstanding alchemists of the time were John Dastin and John of Rupescissa. Dastin was an old-style alchemist absorbed in preparing the Philosopher's Stone; John of Rupescissa, on the other hand, adopted the Lullian theories about the quintessence and played a central role in the evolution of medical alchemy. The creative centuries of Latin alchemy were the thirteenth and fourteenth; in the fifteenth, there was a slackening, and, after that, the rise of modern science caused the adepts to veer more and more towards the completely speculative and mystical Hermetic Philosophy.[116] However, before that transition occurred, much alchemical theory and practice had been taken up by chemistry and medicine.

In Latin alchemy, the most cogent rationale for prolongevitism is found in the writings of Roger Bacon.[117]

---

[109] *Ibid.*, p. 104.
[110] On the Arabic forerunners of the idea of progress, see *ibid.*, pp. 124–126.
[111] *Ibid.*, p. 124.
[112] The best survey of Latin alchemy is Taylor, *Alchemists,* pp. 95–144. Other reliable works are Holmyard, *Alchemy,* pp. 102–148; Lippmann, *op. cit.* (see fn. 1) **1,** part 5 and the relevant sections of Lynn Thorndike, *A History of Magic and Experimental Science* (8 v., New York, 1923 ff.) **2, 3** and **4,** hereafter referred to as "Thorndike, *Magic.*" In addition, there is the book by W. Ganzenmuller, popular in style but based on sound research, *L'Alchimie au moyen âge,* G. Petit-Dutaillis, transl. from German ed. of 1938 (Paderborn), (Paris, n.d.: *ca.* 1940).
[113] Holmyard, *Alchemy,* p. 131.
[114] *Ibid.*, pp. 112–114.

[115] On the relation of Arnald of Villanova to alchemy, see Thorndike, *Magic* **3:** pp. 52–84 and Paul Diepgen, *Medizin und Kultur* (Stuttgart, 1938), pp. 127–149. On Lull and alchemy, see Robert Amadou, *Raymond Lulle et l'alchimie* (Paris ?, 1953), especially pp. 25–31.
[116] On these later phases of alchemy, see Taylor, *Alchemists,* pp. 190–230.
[117] On Roger Bacon's career, useful surveys are Stewart C. Easton, *Roger Bacon and his Search for a Universal Science* (New York, 1952); Thorndike, *Magic* **2:** pp. 616–691; A. G. Little, ed., *Roger Bacon Essays* (Oxford, 1914) and John Henry Bridges, *The Life and Work of Roger Bacon* (London, 1914). See also Dorothea Waley Singer, "Alchemical Writings Attributed to Roger Bacon," *Speculum* **7** (1932): pp. 80–86. The bulk of Bacon's prolongevitist writings are found in the following four works: (1) *Opus majus,* of which I have used the Robert Belle Burke transl. (see fn. 2); hereafter referred to as "Bacon, *Majus.*" (2) *Cure of Old Age, and Preservation of Youth,* Richard Browne, transl. (London, 1683); hereafter referred to as "Bacon, *Cure.*" (3) *De retardatione accidentium senectutis, cum aliis opusculis de rebus medicinalibus,* A. G. Little and E. Withington, eds., British Society of Franciscan Studies **14** (Oxford, 1928); this collection includes most of the material of the Browne translation and a good deal more. (4) *Letter Concerning the Marvelous Power of Art and of Nature,* Tenney L. Davis, transl. (Easton, Pa., London and Tokyo, 1923); hereafter referred to as "Bacon, *Letter.*"

The Oxford scholar presented, in the *Opus majus*, four reasons why, in his own times, the brevity of life must be considered accidental (and subject to improvement) rather than essential (and, therefore, fixed). The first reason reflects the antediluvian theme, that people lived much longer in the past:

At the beginning of the world there was a great prolongation of life, but now it has been shortened unduly.[118]

Bacon was influenced strongly in this direction by Judeo-Christian traditions about Eden and the ten patriarchs.

The possibility of the prolongation of life is confirmed by the consideration that the soul naturally is immortal and capable of not dying. So, after the fall, a man might live for a thousand years [i.e., Methuselah]; and since that time the length of life has been gradually shortened. Therefore it follows that this shortening is accidental and may be remedied wholly or in part.[119]

While Thorndike insists there is no reason to believe that Bacon was persecuted by the Church authorities, it must be admitted that his use of Scripture verges on the unorthodox.

As second and third reasons, Bacon argued that longevity was decreased by widespread immorality and by the neglect of hygiene. Bacon's precept that unethical behavior causes a shortened life span can be deduced logically from the teachings of the Church Fathers, but like many of his other ideas on prolongevitism, it seems closer to the spirit of the Hebrews, and still more to Taoism, than to that of Christianity.

For sins weaken the powers of the soul, so that it is incompetent for the natural control of the body; and therefore the powers of the body are weakened and life is shortened.[120]

Along with sin, the common failure to observe the code of health also weakens the life force.

For although the regimen of health should be observed . . . from infancy, no one wishes to take thought in regard to them, not even physicians. . . . Very rarely does it happen that any one pays sufficient heed to the rules of health. No one does so in his youth, but sometimes one in three thousand thinks of these matters when he is old and approaching death. . . .[121]

The detrimental influence of these factors is compounded with each succeeding generation, for Bacon believed in the inheritance of acquired characteristics.

Therefore fathers are weakened and beget weak sons with a liability to premature death. Then by neglect of the rules of health the sons weaken themselves, and thus the son's son has a doubly weakened constitution. . . . Thus a weakened constitution passes from father to sons, until

a final shortening of life has been reached, as is the case in these days.[122]

As the fourth reason for regarding the life span to be flexible, Bacon asserted there were numerous instances in which individuals, by "secret arts," had added remarkably to their years. In the West, stories of this type performed the same function as the *hsien* literature in China. Bacon's favorite was one about a Sicilian farmer:

. . . in the time of King William of Sicily a man was found who renewed the period of his youth in strength and sense and sagacity beyond all human calculation for about sixty years, and from a rustic ploughman became a messenger of the king. While ploughing he found a golden vessel in the fields hidden in the earth, which contained an excellent liquor. Thinking this liquor was dew from the sky he drank it and washed his face, and was renewed in mind and body beyond measure.[123]

What made this fable so attractive was the implication that the farmer had benefited from a solution of gold; this was in accord with the alchemical quest for potable gold.[124]

Bacon noted many more tales of this sort; among others, there was the English woodsman who anointed his body with a strange ointment and "lived three hundred years without any corruption," there was a captive of the Saracens who obtained "a medicine" which prolonged his life five hundred years, and there was a man who took "a medicine prepared by scientists for a great king" and lived several centuries.[125] Bacon particularly was impressed by the case of "Artephius":

. . . Artephius, who wisely studied the forces of animals, stones, etc., for the purpose of learning the secrets of Nature, especially the secret of the length of life, gloried in living for one thousand and twenty-five years.[126]

This "Artephius" is identified by Thorndike as al-Tughra'i, an Arabic alchemist who died in 1128[127]; strangely enough, Bacon was not troubled by the fact that this sage enjoyed a life span greater than that of any of the Biblical patriarchs.

In Bacon, as in Taoist prolongevitism, one finds traces of each of the standard themes of prolongevity legend. In addition to the antediluvian theme, there are, as we have just seen, numerous variants of the fountain theme, that there exist substances with wondrous powers to lengthen life. The hyperborean theme, that peoples in distant lands have prodigious longevity, is represented by such accounts as those of the Ethi-

---

[118] Bacon, *Majus*, p. 617. *Cf.* earlier, chap. III, section on antediluvian theme.

[119] Bacon, *Letter*, p. 35. For Aquinas' belief that divine grace was necessary for immortality even before the Fall, see earlier, chap. II.

[120] Bacon, *Majus*, p. 618.

[121] *Ibid.*, pp. 617–618.

[122] *Ibid.*, p. 618.

[123] *Ibid.*, p. 622. The fable also appears in Bacon, *Cure*, p. 75, and Bacon, *Letter*, pp. 33–34.

[124] The story is used explicitly to recommend potable gold in Bacon, *Majus*, p. 623. The idea is strikingly similar to the first Chinese reference to alchemy; see earlier, *re* Ssu-ma Ch'ien.

[125] Bacon, *Letter*, p. 34 and *Majus*, p. 622.

[126] Bacon, *Letter*, pp. 34–35.

[127] Thorndike, *Magic* 2: p. 354.

opians, who preserve their youth by eating the flesh of dragons, and the wise men of Chaldea, who "even at this time" rejuvenate themselves by replacing the old moisture of the body with new.[128]

Like Ko Hung, Bacon was fascinated by the phoenix theme, that certain animals are able to avoid aging; however, while the Chinese admired the tortoise and the crane, Bacon singled out the stag, the eagle, and the serpent.[129] Bacon ascribed the longevity of these animals to their instinctive knowledge of the medical powers of herbs and minerals. In support of this thesis, he tells of a Parisian scholar who inflicted grievous wounds on a snake, and then observed the creature seek out a certain herb which effected an immediate cure.[130] As usual, these phoenix-type stories lead to the moral that, if lowly animals can prolong their lives, it is all the more certain that human beings also can do so.[131]

All these considerations moved Bacon to assert that longevity could be extended significantly, and, on this point, he rightly pictured himself as sharply at variance with the customary attitude of Western medicine. Galen and Avicenna (see earlier, chap. II) had had scant sympathy for prolongevity; their regimens were designed to give the aged a moderate degree of protection from disease, but in no way did they attempt to reverse the process of senescence. The tradition had been to protect the aged; Bacon aimed to *free* them.

. . . the things which are laid down by us in this epistle, differ very much from the things laid down by the Ancients. First, because the Ancients' regimen of living defends men's bodies from hastening to their end besides the course of nature; but our regimen lays open by what way old men and the well-stricken in years may easily be freed and defended from the accidents of old age. . . .[132]

Along with his therapeutic activism, the friar developed a more querulous attitude towards aging than the classical physicians. To Galen, old age was not a disease, for it was not contrary to nature; and Galen consequently was tolerant of the "inevitable" infirmities of the senescent. Bacon, in contrast, was more outspoken about the "evils" and "corruption" of old age and his portrayal of senescence is very grim:

. . . excess of mucus, foul phlegm, inflammation of the eyes, and general injury to the organs of sense, diminution of blood and of the spirits, weakness in motion and breathing and in the whole body, failure in both the animal and natural powers of the soul, sleeplessness, anger and disquietude of mind, and forgetfulness. . . .[133]

The Oxford scholar would have had little patience with Cicero's apologist efforts to idealize old age and to envision the elderly devoting themselves to the cultivation of character and the formulation of wise counsel.[134] Such hopes would seem unrealistic to Bacon, who assumed that a sound mind was impossible without a sound body,[135] and who described the aged as sore beset by the simultaneous deterioration of mind, body, and spirit.

Although Bacon surpassed the classical schools of medicine in his aspirations for retarding age, his expectations were not as unbounded as those of the Taoists. The friar was too much circumscribed by the framework of Christian thought to state that men might gain the immortality of a *hsien:* ". . . for there is a limit in Nature, imposed upon the first men after the fall from grace."[136] What he did suggest was that "life might be prolonged a century or more beyond the usual age of men now living."[137] Bacon asserted that, in his own times, old age usually began between forty-five and fifty.[138] Thus, he was thinking in terms of a life span of one hundred and fifty years or more; this would be attainable by members of his own generation, and we may assume that the effect of the inheritance of acquired characteristics might augment this to the three to five centuries which recur in his stories about the prolongation of life.

The two aspects of his work in which Bacon was least original were his theory of the cause of aging and his program of hygiene. He began his book on the preservation of youth with an excellent summary of Avicenna's explanation of senescence.[139] The cause of old age is the loss of "innate" heat, which, in turn, is due to the decay of "innate" moisture and the accumulation of abnormal moisture. This innate moisture is a more ethereal and spiritual principle than any ordinary moisture; it is, in fact, a vitalist concept akin to the "essence" of Taoist biology. The innate moisture produces the innate heat just as oil feeds the flame of a lamp. The reasons given by Bacon to explain the decline of the innate moisture are exactly the same as those noted by Avicenna in his *Canon* of medicine. The difference between the two writers is that Bacon believed the process could be halted or even reversed, the two weapons for the struggle being hygiene and pharmacology.

In the battle against aging, hygiene had far the lesser

[128] Bacon, *Majus*, pp. 623–624 and *Cure*, p. 61. On the prolongevity folklore themes, see earlier, chap. III, and also chap. IV, section on magic and folklore.
[129] Bacon, *Majus*, pp. 620–621 and *Letter*, p. 34.
[130] Bacon, *Majus*, p. 621.
[131] *Idem.*
[132] Bacon, *Cure*, p. 136; the English has been modernized somewhat here.
[133] Bacon, *Majus*, p. 619.

[134] On Cicero, see earlier, chap. II, section on philosophy. It should be stated, on behalf of Cicero's argument, that the elderly in the Roman Republic (as in China) had a rather high status; e.g., the word "senate," derived from the word for aged.
[135] Bacon, *Cure*, p. 40.
[136] Bacon, *Letter*, p. 37.
[137] *Ibid.*, p. 36.
[138] Bacon, *Majus*, p. 619.
[139] Bacon, *Cure*, pp. 2–6; for the hypotheses of Aristotle, Galen, and Avicenna on old age, see earlier, chap. II, section on biology and medicine.

role. Bacon's regimen scarcely deviated from the traditional measures for controlling diet, exercise, breathing, elimination, sexual activity, rest, and the emotions.[140] This was a long but rather easy-going set of rules which Sigerist has termed a hygiene of the leisure class[141]; it was far removed from the ambitious physiological techniques of the Taoists. Bacon always remained ambivalent in his attitude towards hygiene. On the one hand, he felt that it well might promote longevity:

The proper regimen of health, therefore, as far as a man can possess it, would prolong life beyond its common accidental limit, which man because of his folly does not protect for his own interest; and thus some have lived for many years beyond the common limit of life.[142]

But then again, he grew impatient of its impractical nature:

For who can avoid the air infected with putrid vapors carried about with the force of the winds? Who will measure out meat and drink? Who can weigh in a sure scale or degree sleep and watching, motion and rest and things that vanish in a moment, and the accidents of the mind, so that they shall neither exceed nor fall short?[143]

To replenish the "innate" moisture, Bacon placed his chief hope on pharmacology, or

. . : the knowledge of those properties, that are in certain things, which the ancients have kept secret.[144]

Like Ko Hung, Bacon listed a number of substances with marvelous powers of rejuvenation: pearls, coral, rosemary, aloe wood, the flesh of serpents, ambergris, gold and the bone from a stag's heart.[145] Nearly all these drugs had been praised by previous medical writers[146]; what was novel and "secret" about Bacon's attitude was the fact that he assessed them from the alchemical standpoint, according to which everything in the world possesses a greater or less amount of vitalized principle akin to the vital spirit (or innate moisture) of living things.[147]

I have also found this, that there is an admirable virtue placed in plants, animals and stones: which is partly hidden from the men of this age. . . .[148]

We have here, then, a Latin counterpart to the *hsien* medicines of the Chinese, and it is easy to see that the appealing features of these substances were similar to those cited by Ko Hung. Serpents and the stag were supposedly long-lived animals and, therefore, must possess some prolongevity quality. Ambergris, aloe wood, and rosemary would be esteemed for their attractive fragrance; one is reminded of the perfumed life-restoring waters described by Herodotus.[149] Coral was a sort of living mineral, as was pearl which possessed a beauty and lustre that had won it a place among the *hsien* medicines. In choosing these prolongevity drugs, the guiding dictum was that the vital principle from external sources will augment that of the human body.

In like manner, because of similitude, let the square stone of the noble animal [bone from a stag's heart], the mineral sun [gold], and the matter which swims in the sea [coral] be made use of. These three things well prepared are assimilated to the native heat of a healthy man.[150]

One of the most highly esteemed, and certainly the most unusual, of Bacon's remedies was the breath of a young virgin, an item which was believed to meet the criteria of therapy based on analogy; for a youth would have a great store of the vital principle, some of which could be imparted to others in the immediate vicinity. Just as disease was known to be contagious, so also health was believed to be capable of transmission to others through the air or by physical contact. ". . . the infirmity of a man passeth into man; and so doth health because of likeness."[151] The Franciscan scholar discussed this topic in the most circumspect terms, using all sorts of veiled language and warning of the danger of misinterpretation by incontinent persons.[152] Actually, the inspiration for the idea came directly from the Old Testament (I Kings 1: 1–4), in which it is related how the aged King David was warmed by lying abed with a beautiful maiden, with whom, it is stated, he did not have sexual intercourse. The idea was still extant in the seventeenth and eighteenth centuries; it was recommended covertly by Sydenham and Boerhaave and popularized by a half-serious, half-jesting work by Cohausen entitled *Hermippus redivivus,* in honor of Hermippus, a Roman alleged to have prolonged his life in this way.[153]

The Latin alchemists, like the Chinese, singled out gold for special praise as a vitalizing agent. John Dastin, for example, glorified the noble metal in the same terms used by Wei Po-yang and Ko Hung; it was not diminished by fire, and it was not corroded by air, earth, or water.[154] Being incorruptible itself, this "mineral sun," by the rule of analogy, must be able

[140] *Ibid.,* pp. 53 ff. *Cf.* Robert Montraville Green, transl., *Galen's Hygiene: De sanitate tuenda* (Springfield, Ill., 1951).
[141] Henry E. Sigerist, *Landmarks in the History of Hygiene* (London, 1956), pp. 13–14.
[142] Bacon, *Majus,* p. 620.
[143] Bacon, *Cure,* pp. 13–14.
[144] *Ibid.,* p. 11.
[145] *Ibid.,* pp. 15–16 and *Majus,* p. 623.
[146] Little, *op. cit.* (see fn. 117), p. 351.
[147] Bacon stated that alchemy should guide medicine in the choice and preparation of drugs; Bacon, *De retardatione* (see fn. 117), pp. 155–158.
[148] Bacon, *Cure,* pp. 46–47.

[149] See earlier, chap. III, section on the fountain theme.
[150] Bacon, *Cure,* p. 103.
[151] *Ibid.,* p. 100.
[152] *Ibid.,* pp. 99–103 and *De retardatione* (see fn. 117), pp. 140–142.
[153] Mirko D. Grmek, *On Ageing and Old Age: Basic Problems and Historic Aspects of Gerontology and Geriatrics,* Monographiae biologicae 5, 2 (Den Haag, 1958), pp. 44–45.
[154] John Dastin, "Letter to Pope John XXII," C. H. Josten, transl., *Ambix* 4 (1949): pp. 45–46. Also on Dastin, see Thorndike, *Magic* 3: pp. 85–102.

to impart its characteristics to man; as Bacon puts it, "For that preserves another thing which is long preserved itself. . . ."[155] From this, it followed that gold would be an admirable medicine for preventing age, as we read already in the Latin Geber: "Also gold is of metals the most precious . . . (it) is a medicine rejoicing, and conserving the body in youth.[156]

According to Arnald of Villanova, the action of gold, which he called "a miracle of nature," was to cleanse and clear the substance of the heart,[157] traditionally the seat of the innate moisture.[158] One of the attractions of alchemy was the dream of preparing artificial gold of a higher quality than the natural variety; in the words of Bacon,

. . . experimental science . . . knows how to produce gold not only of twenty-four degrees [carats] but of thirty and forty degrees and of as many degrees as we desire.[159]

The Sicilian ploughman, hero of Bacon's favorite story, had rejuvenated himself by drinking a solution of this superior sort of gold.[160] Like their Taoist predecessors, the Latin alchemists were much concerned with methods of preparing potable gold, one of the simplest and most direct procedures being that of Arnald of Villanova, who quenched red-hot gold leaf in wine.[161]

Far more precious than gold, however, was the elixir or philosopher's stone which perfected everything in its own kind: base metals were transmuted to silver and gold, while the ill and the aged were restored to health and youth. In the words of John Dastin,

This is the secret of secrets . . . concerning the most noble matter [the philosopher's stone] which, according to the tradition of all philosophers, transforms any metallic body into very pure gold and silver, which conserves (bodies in their) essence, fortifies (them) in (their) virtue, which makes an old man young and drives out all sickness of the body.[162]

The preparation of this stone involved an almost interminable series of chemical manipulations—distillations, dissolvings, precipitations, burnings, and heatings in which the essential material was a specially prepared "mercury"; the clearest picture of the operations involved may be obtained from the handbook compiled by the Latin Geber.[163]

In Bacon's theory of the elixir, there was an echo of the principle of the balance originated by the Arabic Jabir:

If the elements should be prepared and purified in some mixture, so that there would be no action of one element on another, but so that they would be reduced to pure simplicity, the wisest have judged that they would have the most perfect medicine. For in this way the elements would be equal.[164]

Following this, the friar proceeded in characteristic manner to skate a semi-heretical figure eight over some very thin ice:

For this condition will exist in our bodies after the resurrection. For an equality of elements in those bodies excludes corruption for ever. . . . The body of Adam did not possess elements in full equality. . . but since the elements in him approached equality, there was very little waste in him; and hence he was fit for immortality, which he could have secured if he had eaten always of the fruit of the tree of life. For this fruit is thought to have elements approaching equality. . . . Scientists, therefore, have striven to reduce the elements in some form of food or drink to an equality or nearly so, and have taught the means to this end.[165]

In other words, the philosopher's stone is likened to the forbidden fruit of the tree of life (guarded by an angel with flaming sword!),[166] and it seems that the Franciscan came close to the concept of immortality of the sort enunciated earlier by Ko Hung and to be envisioned later by Condorcet. However, the Latin alchemist did not carry this tendency to logical, and possibly heretical, conclusions.

The most original and significant contribution of Latin alchemy was the idea that man could gain control of the fifth element or quintessence.[167] In the cosmology of Aristotle, the fifth element had been far beyond human reach: all the objects and beings of the earth were composed of the ordinary four elements and were subject to generation and decay, while the home of the divine quintessence was the heavens, where it endowed the stars with beauty and immortality. Already in Roman times, however, this sharp distinction between the terrestrial and celestial spheres had become partly blurred, first by the Stoics with their materialization of spirit, and then by the Neoplatonists with their spiritualization of matter. Moreover, much of ancient and medieval alchemy had been based on the semi-pantheist concept that all things contain an ethereal principle allied to life, spirit, and the divine.

The unidentified authors of the Lullian corpus, in the early fourteenth century, were the first to identify this alchemical "virtue" or "spirit" with the Aristotelian quintessence. According to Lullian precepts, God made the world of a "mercury," the grosser part of which

[155] Bacon, Cure, p. 17.
[156] Geber, op. cit. (see fn. 86), p. 64.
[157] Walter Pagel, Paracelsus: an Introduction to Philosophical Medicine in the Era of the Renaissance (Basel and New York, 1958), p. 256; this work hereafter is referred to as "Pagel, Paracelsus."
[158] E.g., Bacon, Cure, p. 6.
[159] Bacon, Majus, p. 627.
[160] Ibid., p. 626.
[161] Henry E. Sigerist, transl. and ed., The Earliest Printed Book on Wine (New York, 1943), pp. 36–37.
[162] Dastin, op. cit. (see fn. 154), pp. 43–44.
[163] Geber, op. cit. (see fn. 86).

[164] Bacon, Majus, p. 624.
[165] Ibid., pp. 624–625.
[166] Genesis 3: 24; cf. earlier, chap. II, section on myth and legend.
[167] On the quintessence in alchemy, see Taylor, Alchemists, pp. 110 ff.; F. Sherwood Taylor, "The Idea of the Quintessence," in Edgar A. Underwood, ed., Science, Medicine, and History: Essays in Honour of Charles Singer (2v., London, 1953) 1: pp. 247–265; and Pagel, Paracelsus, pp. 99–100, especially fn. 264.

formed the earthly four elements, while the more subtle fraction was the fifth element, most of which made up the starry sphere, but some of which *remained* in every terrestrial thing. Another important writer on the quintessence, during the fourteenth century, was the Franciscan John of Rupescissa, who referred to it as an incorruptible virtue conferred by God upon Nature.[168] This fifth element could be extracted by human artifice, he wrote, and could work marvelous cures. While he ruled out any hope of immortality, considering the fall of man from grace, he did think it possible that one might remain youthful until the very hour of death appointed by God.

This new theory of the quintessence seems to have stemmed directly from the discovery of alcohol.[169] The alchemists long had practiced the distillation of various substances, and wine, being an important medicine at the time, was naturally one of the substances tested. However, because the distillation of alcohol required a rather complex technical knowledge, it was not until about 1100 that the effort was successful.[170] To the alchemists, its properties appeared almost incredible: it was a "water" (liquid) and yet it was combustible; it was both cool (to the touch) and warm (to the taste); animal flesh placed in it was preserved from decomposition; and its effects on the human spirit are well known. Alcohol concentrated enough to burn was named *aqua ardens* and, during the thirteenth century, was recommended widely as a valuable medicine; indeed, it was not until the sixteenth century that it began to be used more lightly. It soon was learned that still finer distillates could be obtained, and these were termed *aqua vitae*. In the fourteenth century, the Lullian school postulated that an ultrarefined fraction of this *aqua vitae* would be identical with the quintessence.

Having got hold of a "quintessence" of wine, the alchemists next attempted to isolate the quintessences of other substances.[171] Alcohol being an excellent solvent for a host of organic compounds, their experiments led to the extraction, from herbs, of medicines more powerful than those previously known. This fact was reported in the work of John of Rupescissa, but the friar's mind was dominated too much by the alchemical heritage to follow through on this insight. To Rupescissa, as to nearly all previous alchemists (Jabir is an exception), the best medicines were to be obtained from the mineral kingdom, and he grew most enthusiastic over quintessences of that sort, which were isolated by means of acid treatments. Antimony, for example,

was dissolved in vinegar (acetic acid) and the solution was concentrated into "ruby drops like blood."

Which blessed liquor keep by itself in a strong glass bottle tightly sealed, because it is a treasure which the whole world cannot equal. . . . For all men have toiled to sublimate the spirits of minerals and never had the fifth essence of the aforesaid antimony. . . . it takes away pain from wounds and heals marvelously. Its virtue is incorruptible, miraculous, and useful beyond measure.[172]

In addition to the quintessences of wine and of antimony, Rupescissa also highly valued those of mercury and gold.

CONCLUSION

It now is recognized that the work of Rupescissa marks the transition from alchemy to medical chemistry (iatrochemistry).[173] The iatrochemists differed from the alchemists in having little, if any, concern for the transmutation of base metals into precious ones; their interest was rather in explaining the human body in chemical terms and seeking cures by chemical means. And while the iatrochemists were not averse to speculating about an elixir of youth, the bulk of their attention was devoted to finding specific remedies for specific diseases. Rupescissa's interpretation of the quintessence had shattered the oversimplified scheme of alchemy, for no longer was there only one elixir or quintessence but an innumerable host of quintessences; each substance in the world had a fifth essence of its own with its individual characteristics. This trend towards complexity and sophistication was furthered by Paracelsus, who, in opposition to the general, humoral pathology of Galen, propounded the *specificity* of disease, and, consequently, the need for a multitude of individual, specific remedies.[174]

With Paracelsus, alchemy had come to the end of the road; however, it should not be overlooked that in his work there are noteworthy influences from the alchemical tradition.[175] From childhood, Paracelsus had been deeply interested in alchemy.[176] With the alchemists, he sought the "virtues" in things, the fifth essences, which he considered supernatural emanations from God.[177] Like the Taoists, he considered "prime"

[168] On John of Rupescissa, see Thorndike, *Magic* 3: pp. 347–369; Pagel, *Paracelsus*, pp. 264–265; and Multhauf, *op. cit.* (see fn. 12).

[169] On alcohol and the quintessence, see Taylor, *Alchemists*, pp. 117–121; Pagel, *Paracelsus*, p. 264.

[170] On the discovery of alcohol, see R. J. Forbes, *Short History of the Art of Distillation* (Leiden, 1948), pp. 87–98.

[171] Taylor, *Alchemists*, pp. 120–121.

[172] Thorndike, *Magic* 3: p. 360.

[173] On the transition from alchemy to iatrochemistry, see Multhauf, *op. cit.* (see fn. 12) and his two other articles, "Medical Chemistry and 'the Paracelsans'" and "The Significance of Distillation in Renaissance Medical Chemistry," *Bull. Hist. Medicine* 28 (1954): pp. 101–126 and 30 (1956): pp. 329–346; also Pagel, *Paracelsus*, pp. 241–278 and Taylor, *Alchemists*, pp. 190–201.

[174] Pagel, *Paracelsus*, pp. 129–130, 142.

[175] The best available work on the medical reformer, and a superb piece of intellectual and cultural history, is Pagel, *Paracelsus*; with it, one may use the lucid biography by Henry M. Pachter, *Magic into Science: the Story of Paracelsus* (New York, 1951). The enormous literature on Paracelsus is surveyed in Pagel, *Paracelsus*, pp. 31–35.

[176] Pagel, *Paracelsus*, p. 8.

[177] *Ibid.*, pp. 54–56.

matter as living, incomprehensible, the mother of all things, evolving towards "ultimate" or perfected matter.[178] His system was founded on likenesses between the macrocosm and the microcosm; he spoke, for example, of the minerals in the heart of the earth evolving towards the noble gold, emeralds, and coral, which in turn were useful in strengthening and ennobling the heart of man.[179] Like Ko Hung, he chose medicines according to the doctrine of "signatures" and analogies, and he was fascinated by the problem of the prolongation of life.[180] Indeed, one well might refer to Paracelsus as the last of the great alchemists, and, at the same time, the first of the great iatrochemists. For if Rupescissa was the initiator of medical chemistry, it was the revolutionary Paracelsus who made it an attractive and formidable system and directed it on the path which ultimately was to lead to modern biochemistry and chemotherapy.[181]

VII. THE HYGIENISTS [1]

Lewis Cornaro was an extraordinary and admirable Instance of Long Life; for he lived a hundred Years without any Decay in his Health or Understanding. By his Temperance and the Regimen he observed, he recovered his Constitution from some infirmities, the Liberty of his Youth had brought upon him. . . . He wrote Books on this Argument in his Old Age, in which he . . . promises himself a great many Years to come: Neither was he deceived in his Expectation; for he held out above a Hundred, and then died a very easy Death.

De Thou, *History of His Own Time* [2]

---

[178] *Ibid.*, pp. 91–92, 106, 112–113.
[179] *Ibid.*, pp. 65 ff., 109.
[180] On signatures, *ibid.*, pp. 148–149; on the prolongation of life, see, in Arthur Edward Waite, transl., *The Hermetic and Alchemical Writings of Paracelsus* (2 v., London, 1894), such treatises as "A Book Concerning Long Life" 2: pp. 108 ff. and "The Book Concerning Renovation and Restoration" 2: pp. 124 ff.
[181] On the contribution of Paracelsus to iatrochemistry, see Pagel, *Paracelsus,* pp. 273–278 and the studies by Allen G. Debus, "The Paracelsian Aerial Niter," *Isis* **55** (1964): pp. 43–61 and *The English Paracelsians* (London, 1965).
[1] I have not seen any monograph dealing specifically with prolongevity hygiene. A gracious introduction to the history of general hygiene is Henry E. Sigerist, *Landmarks in the History of Hygiene* (London, 1956). On codes of hygiene for the aged and for lengthening life, there is information scattered through Mirko D. Grmek, "On Ageing and Old Age: Basic Problems and Historic Aspects of Gerontology and Geriatrics." *Monographiae biologicae* 5, 2 (Den Haag, 1958) and Frederic D. Zeman, "Life's Later Years: Studies in the Medical History of Old Age," *Jour. Mt. Sinai Hospital* (N. Y.); for vols. and pp., see later, Bibliography. There is a sketchy article by Sona Rosa Burstein, "The 'Cure' of Old Age: Codes of Health," *Geriatrics* **10** (1955): pp. 328–332. Many early works on hygiene are listed under "Early Discussions Before 1900" in Nathan W. Shock, *A Classified Bibliography of Gerontology and Geriatrics* (Stanford, Calif., 1951) and *Supplement One: 1949–1955* (1957).
[2] Quoted in the translator's preface to Leonard Lessius, *Hygiasticon,* Timothy Smith, transl. (London, 1742). *Cf.* Jacques Auguste de Thou, *Histoire universelle,* A. F. Prévost, P. F. Guyot *et al.,* transl. (London, 1734), book 38 in **5**: pp. 122–123.

LUIGI CORNARO

It is ironic that Jacob Burckhardt, in his endeavor to portray the uniqueness of the Italian Renaissance as the precursor of modern culture, failed to assess adequately the significance of Luigi Cornaro. In speaking of the effect which the revival of antiquity had on Italian literature, he mentioned the "classical perfection" of Cornaro's style.[3] Later, in discussing the new type of biographical work introduced by the Renaissance, he selected four remarkable autobiographies: those of Pius II, Cellini, Cardano and, "one man who was both worthy and happy," Cornaro. He quoted several long extracts from the *Vita sobria,* and these give a vivid picture of Cornaro's personality and his manner of life.[4] One receives an impression of a man who found life vastly interesting and enjoyable, a man who expressed himself easily and gracefully and with an almost childlike candor. But Cornaro's views on the prolongation of life were neglected, although this is the aspect of his work which supports most strongly Burckhardt's thesis that

. . . it was not the revival of antiquity alone, but its union with the genius of the Italian people, which achieved the conquest of the western world. . . . The Renaissance is not a mere fragmentary imitation or compilation, but a new birth.[5]

Cornaro's *Discorsi della vita sobria* meets almost exactly Burckhardt's criteria for a typical production of the Renaissance: a number of Greco-Roman ideas are combined in a novel way and are infused with a modern spirit. The ideas of Cornaro were derived from Cicero and Galen, but his interpretation of them differed from that of antiquity. Cicero, in his *De senectute,* had attempted to idealize old age, but his purpose was apologist, and, consequently, the mood of his treatise was rather defensive, like that of a lawyer saddled with a guilty client.[6] Galen in *De sanitate tuenda* had formulated a complex system of hygiene for the leisure class, but his aim was very limited; he had little enthusiasm for either old age or the prolongation of life.[7] What Cornaro did was to take Cicero's views and use them to argue the *desirability* of prolongevity. Galen's regime he simplified and popularized; and, at the same time, he made unprecedented claims for its effectiveness, so as to support the *possibility* of prolongevity. The entire tone of Cornaro's narrative, his optimism and zest for living, is in marked contrast to comparable Classical writings.[8]

---

[3] Jacob Burckhardt, *The Civilization of the Renaissance,* S. G. C. Middlemore, transl. (London and New York, 1944), p. 145.
[4] *Ibid.*, pp. 204–206.
[5] *Ibid.*, pp. 104, 106.
[6] On Cicero, see earlier, chap. II, section on philosophy.
[7] On Galen, see earlier, chap. II, section on biology and medicine.
[8] *Cf.* Epicurean and Stoic ideas about longevity; see earlier, chap. II, section on philosophy.

In nearly every respect, Cornaro was a typical member of the Italian nobility during the era of the Renaissance.[9] The Cornaro family, like many others, was caught up in the political life of the city-states of Northern Italy, and consequently its members were subjected to violent changes of fortune. The interests of the family were centered in Venice, but Cornaro's grandfather, having been banished from that city, had settled in Padua; there Luigi was born in 1467.[10] By shrewd management of his lands, Cornaro became very wealthy and was able to restore the patent of nobility which had been lost in the Venetian intrigues. In the manner of the time, he was a lavish patron of the arts, especially architecture, and his homes and villas were widely admired; one of them, for example, included decorations by Raphael. As was customary, Cornaro did not confine himself to business and politics but also designed buildings, initiated public works and even wrote a gay comedy. During the 1530's and 1540's, he was a member of the Paduan circle of Bembo, the distinguished humanist, and there he was acquainted with Fracastoro, the poet-physician.

The most appealing feature of the *Vita sobria,* and one which must have gained for it numerous readers, is the success story which serves as its *raison d'être,* a success measured not in terms of income or fame but in health and longevity.[11] According to Cornaro, between the ages of thirty-five and forty he had found his constitution utterly ruined by a disorderly way of life and by frequent overindulgence in sensual pleasures.[12] Among other things, he was suffering from pains in the stomach and side, gout, fever, and an insatiate thirst; his condition had deteriorated to such an extent as to call forth the warning of physicians that, without a drastic reform in his habits, he could survive but a few months more. It was in these desperate circumstances, we are told, that he adopted that temperate and orderly life, of which he was to be the most popular exponent. Following this almost religious conversion, Cornaro rapidly recovered and retained his well-being throughout the middle years and far into old age. In 1550, at the age of eighty-three, Cornaro, at the request of his younger friends, composed the first *Discourse*

propounding his regimen of health; the second discourse was added at the age of eighty-six, the third at ninety-one and the fourth at ninety-five. According to Maroncelli, the wise patriarch passed away in 1565 at the age of ninety-eight.[13]

Cornaro presented four arguments, all more or less novel, in favor of the desirability of longevity. Of these, the first is a simple affirmation of the worth of long life. Not only did he casually refer to Nature as "being desirous to preserve man as long as possible," but he also thought of God in the same light [14]:

Our Maker, having ordained that the life of man should last for many years, is desirous that everyone should attain the extreme limit; since He knows that, after the age of eighty, man is wholly freed from the bitter fruits of sensuality. . . . Then, of necessity, vices and sins are left behind. Wherefore it is that God wishes we should all live to extreme age.[15]

This is much closer to the spirit of Cicero than to Paul, yet the venerable Paduan regarded himself a very good Christian. It was, however, a sort of Christianity far removed from the temper of the Middle Ages, for Cornaro felt he could have the best of both this world and the next.

. . . in this extreme age of mine [ninety-five], I enjoy two lives at the same time: one, the earthly, which I possess in reality; the other, the heavenly, which I possess in thought.[16]

Nor was Cornaro impressed by the mortification of the flesh sought by medieval saints as reparation for their sins:

I cannot refrain from saying that, according to my judgment, these persons are mistaken; for I cannot believe God deems it good that man, whom He so much loves, should be sickly, melancholy, and discontented. I believe, on the contrary, that He wishes him to be healthy, cheerful, and contented. . . .[17]

Where Paul scarcely could persuade himself to continue his earthly existence, the choice was made by Cornaro with irrepressible zeal: ". . . I ceaselessly keep repeating, Live, live, that you may become better servants of God!"[18]

The second reason for the desirability of longevity is that old age is a happy phase of life, an argument which represented a departure from traditional Western prolongevitism. Most previous advocates of long life had thought of prolongevity as virtually synonymous with rejuvenation. Roger Bacon, for example, sought to "cure" old age, and, viewing senescence as an enemy, he did not hesitate to picture it in grim

[9] On Cornaro's life and work, see William B. Walker, "Luigi Cornaro, a Renaissance Writer on Personal Hygiene," *Bull. Hist. Medicine* 28 (1954): pp. 525–534; Piero Maroncelli, "Biography of Alvise [Luigi] Cornaro" in John Burdell, ed., *The Discourses and Letters of Louis Cornaro: on a Sober and Temperate Life* (New York, 1842), pp. 127–153; and Sigerist, *op. cit.* (see fn. 1), pp. 36–46.

[10] The facts regarding the place and date of Cornaro's birth vary in different accounts of his life; according to Walker, the most reliable study is that of Maroncelli, and I here follow his version.

[11] Luigi Cornaro, *Discourses on the Temperate Life,* in William F. Butler, ed., *The Art of Living Long* (Milwaukee, 1903), pp. 37–113; this work is hereafter referred to as "Cornaro, *Discourses.*"

[12] On Cornaro's illness and his recovery through temperance, see *ibid.,* pp. 42–47.

[13] Maroncelli, *op. cit.* (see fn. 9), pp. 143–144.
[14] Cornaro, *Discourses,* p. 61.
[15] *Ibid.,* p. 98.
[16] *Ibid.,* p. 110.
[17] *Ibid.,* p. 112.
[18] *Ibid.,* p. 113. On Paul, see earlier, chap. II, section on New Testament.

terms.[19] The glorification of old age, on the other hand, had been identified with apologism in Cicero's *De senectute*. Now Cornaro adapted the idealization of age to serve the cause of moderate prolongevitism, writing at the age of eighty-three,

And now, since some sensual and unreasonable men pretend . . . that the existence of a man after he has passed the age of sixty-five cannot any longer be called a living life, but rather should be termed a dead one, I shall plainly show that they are much mistaken; for I have an ardent desire that every man should strive to attain my age, in order that he may enjoy . . . the most beautiful period of life.[20]

Cornaro then described with infectious enthusiasm the healthy state of his body and mind[21]; he claimed that, despite his advanced years, his senses were in perfect condition, his disposition was cheerful and contented, he was able to mount his horse unassisted and climb stairs easily, and, perhaps most surprising of all, his teeth remained well preserved. He also wrote eagerly of the joys of his way of life: his reading and writing, his conversations with scholars and artists, his lovely homes and gardens in Padua and in the country, his projects for the reclamation of waste lands, his travels, and, closest to his heart, the company of his eleven grandchildren.

After the disarming *joie de vivre* of his first two arguments, Cornaro moved on to an unexpectedly shrewd and calculating one. Pointing to those who exclaimed that a short, tempestuous life is better than a long, sombre one, he cautioned,

They do not pause to consider what immense importance ten years more of life, and especially of healthy life, possess when we have reached mature age, the time, indeed, at which men appear to the best advantage in learning and virtue—two things which can never reach their perfection except with time.[22]

In support of this assertion, Cornaro remarked that many of the most celebrated works in science and literature were composed in advanced years, and he added, with unconcealed satisfaction, that his own treatises might be mentioned in that regard. In sum, he seems to be saying that longevity pays:

. . . men endowed with fine talents ought to prize a long life very highly . . . a refined and talented man . . . if he is already a cardinal, when he has passed the age of eighty he will the more likely become pope; if he is a public official, how much greater is the possibility of his being called to the highest dignity in the state; if a man of letters, he will be looked upon as a god on earth; and the same is true of all others, according to their various occupations.[23]

Cornaro's originality is demonstrated again in the fourth reason why prolongevity is desirable: if one

lives long enough, he will attain the blessing of a "natural death." The concept of "natural death" was far from new; in Aristotle, the distinction already was made between death from forcible *extinction* (of the innate heat) and death from gradual *exhaustion* (of the innate heat).[24] The former process was identified with disease or physical violence; the latter, comparatively gentle in character, was thought of as natural and was associated with senescence. Cornaro's innovation was to use this idea as an argument for prolongevitism; for, those who, through the practice of temperance, reach an extreme old age will not suffer the agonies which accompany the "unnatural" death of earlier periods of life.

And the inevitable approach of death grieves them so much the less in that it does not come suddenly or unexpectedly, with a troublesome and bitter alteration of the humors, and with sharp pains and cruel fever; but it comes most quietly and mildly. For, in them, the end is caused merely by the failure of the radical ["innate"] moisture; which, consumed by degrees, finally becomes completely exhausted, after the manner of a lamp which gradually fails. Hence they pass away peacefully, and without any kind of sickness. . . .[25]

This notion recurs in various forms in later works on prolongevitism; Metchnikoff, for example, reasoned that, if life could be prolonged greatly enough, death would lose its terrors, because the "instinct of death" gradually would overcome the instinct of self-preservation.[26]

Turning from the desirability of long life to its possibility, we find Cornaro to be a moderate prolongevitist; in comparison with the radical views of the Taoists and the alchemists, he seems almost timorous. Nevertheless, the Italian nobleman was quite firm in extending the life span beyond the "three score and ten or at most four score" of the Bible (Psalms 90: 10); he believed that any person, even one handicapped by a delicate constitution, could live to the age of a hundred, while those endowed with a strong constitution could aspire to one hundred twenty years.[27] What especially classifies Cornaro as a prolongevitist is his opinion that *anyone* may enjoy a life of one hundred to one hundred twenty years. In Greco-Roman tradition, there were instances of remarkable longevity, but these were restricted to exceptionally hardy individuals[28]; Cornaro, however, opened the way for a general prolongation of life.

[19] On Roger Bacon's description of senescence, see earlier, chap. VI, section on Latin alchemy.

[20] Cornaro, *Discourses*, p. 66.

[21] *Ibid.*, pp. 66–72, 92–93.

[22] *Ibid.*, p. 59.

[23] *Ibid.*, p. 84.

[24] Aristotle, *De iuventute et senectute*, G. R. T. Ross, transl. in W. D. Ross and J. A. Smith, eds., *The Works of Aristotle, Translated into English* (12 v., Oxford, [1908–1952] 3: p. 469b.

[25] Cornaro, *Discourses*, p. 65; see also, pp. 73–74, 80, 107. On innate heat and innate moisture, see earlier, chap. II, section on biology and medicine.

[26] Élie Metchnikoff, *The Nature of Man: Studies in Optimistic Philosophy* (New York, 1906), pp. 262 ff.

[27] Cornaro, *Discourses*, pp. 78, 106.

[28] What is meant here are cases of longevity in the native land and in the times of the writers concerned; that is, we are not referring to material of the antediluvian or hyperborean types.

This, certainly a most desirable lot, is one, that will be granted to all, of what degree or condition soever, who lead the temperate life, whether they occupy a high position, or that of the middle class, or are found in the humblest ranks of life; for we all belong to one species, and are composed of the same four elements.[29]

Moreover, this long life, as we have seen, will be healthy and happy to the very end.

The keystone of Cornaro's regimen, of course, was temperance, especially in regard to diet. He attributed his health and longevity to,

. . . these two very important rules which I have always so carefully observed, relative to eating and drinking, namely, to take only the the quantity which my stomach can easily digest and only the kinds that agree with it. . . .[30]

As one matured, it was absolutely essential to reduce the amount of food taken in, because the "natural heat" (i.e., innate heat) decreased in the elderly, and, therefore, they required little food (as fuel).[31] Cornaro also learned from experience that one must be wary in the kinds of food one chooses to eat, for those which appealed to his taste were not always suitable to his digestion. In time, his diet came to consist of small portions of bread, meat, broth with egg, and "new" wine[32]; despite this simple fare, he claimed that, "I always eat with relish," and "I feel, when I leave the table, that I must sing."[33] Along with temperance in diet, it also was helpful, though not essential, to be moderate and orderly in all other things, to guard against great heat or cold, fatigue, melancholy, hatred, and other debilitating influences.[34] In view of his success with this method, the hygienist concluded that, "a man can have no better doctor than himself, and no better medicine than the temperate life."[35]

Cornaro's regimen aimed at prolonging life by conserving the "innate moisture" or vital principle of the body.[36] Unlike the Taoists and the alchemists, he did not envisage any process by which the innate moisture could be restored or increased, thereby causing rejuvenation and a radical increase in longevity. His hopes were more limited: every individual is born with a certain amount of innate moisture which gradually is used up by the body's activities. As this principle of life is consumed, it cannot be regained, but, by leading a temperate life, one may determine that the supply will last for the time allotted to man by God and Nature, one hundred to one hundred twenty years. The major obstacle on the road to long life is disease,

for when one is ill, the innate moisture is expended at an abnormally rapid rate. Cornaro claimed that the great usefulness of his regimen is that it keeps the four humors of the body nicely balanced and, therefore, prevents all disease: ". . . it is impossible, in the regular course of nature that he who leads the orderly and temperate life should ever fall sick."[37] And it follows that

. . . sobriety . . . is more conducive to the preservation of the radical [innate] moisture. . . . Hence we may reasonably conclude that the holy temperate life is the true mother of health and of longevity.[38]

THE CORNARO TRADITION

The *Discourses* gained a wide and enthusiastic audience.[39] The first section of the work had appeared in Italian in 1558; it was translated into Latin in 1613, into English in 1634 and, before the end of the seventeenth century, into French, German, and Dutch. The warmest reception was in England, where in 1711 it received the endorsement of Joseph Addison in *The Spectator*[40]; an idea of its popularity there is suggested by the fact that one English version, during the eighteenth and nineteenth centuries, went through fifty editions. Moreover, the treatises stimulated the production of a host of similar works, all more or less founded on the idea propounded by Cornaro: that longevity can be extended significantly by simple reforms in the individual's habits of life.

A hallmark of the Cornaro tradition is the assumption that a few elementary hygienic practices will have a major effect on one's health; the basis for this belief is an interesting combination of primitivism, individualism, and humoralist pathology. The primitivist element is a sort of precursor of Rousseau's dictum: man is born free but found everywhere in chains; for the hygienists, man is born healthy but found everywhere in ill health. Where Rousseau was to argue that man is *good* by nature and would be virtuous if liberated from excessive institutional controls, the hygienists assumed that man is *healthy* by nature and would no longer be subject to disease if he led a simple and moderate life. There is a large measure of individualism in this, for, if God and Nature have endowed man with health, there is little need for organized medicine; as Cornaro reasoned, "a man can have no better doctor than himself."[41] All this blended rather well with a popularized version of Galenic pathology in which disease represents an imbalance in the humors of the body. Before the day of bacteriology, with its terrifying hordes of invisible microbes, and pathological

[29] Cornaro, *Discourses*, p. 80.
[30] *Ibid.*, p. 48.
[31] *Ibid.*, pp. 105–106.
[32] On Cornaro's diet, see Sigerist, *op. cit.* (see fn. 1), pp. 41–42.
[33] Cornaro, *Discourses*, pp. 87, 107.
[34] *Ibid.*, p. 48.
[35] *Ibid.*, p. 58.
[36] This analysis is based on *ibid.*, pp. 63–65, 78–79, 85, 106–107.

[37] *Ibid.*, p. 106.
[38] *Ibid.*, p. 85.
[39] The various translations and editions of the *Discourses* are discussed in Walker, *op. cit.* (see fn. 9), pp. 530–533 and Sigerist, *op. cit.* (see fn. 1), pp. 45–46.
[40] *The Spectator*, October 13, 1711.
[41] Cornaro, *Discourses*, p. 58.

anatomy, with its insidious and relentless morbid processes in the tissues and cells, it was still possible to envision the control of disease by means of very simple measures.

Another contributing factor in the acceptance of Cornaro-type regimens was the widespread credulity about the human life span. There still was general belief in the antediluvian and hyperborean themes, that people in the past or in other parts of the world enjoyed remarkable longevity; indeed, there was a tendency to accept such accounts even when the cases were located in one's own time and country. A prime example is William Harvey's report on the autopsy of Thomas Parr: Harvey represented the most advanced scientific thought of his time, yet he wrote in a matter-of-fact manner that Parr had reached the age of "one hundred and fifty-two years and nine months." [42] The report also demonstrates the climate of opinion which favored Cornaro's ideas; Harvey attributed the longevity of Parr to the poor farmer's meagre diet, his being "free from care" and his breathing the country air of "perfect purity"; moreover, even at this incredible age, death actually was premature, for it seemed to have been caused by Parr's visit to London with its foul air and rich, complicated foods. These naive views regarding longevity gave added attraction to prolongevity hygiene, for Cornaro had asserted it to be possible for the average person to live out the *full* span of life allotted "by God and Nature." He himself had set the life span at the comparatively modest figure of 120, but there was no reason why others might not extend this to the 152 years of Parr or even beyond that.

Our purpose here is limited to outlining the characteristic ideas of prolongevity hygiene; to that end, we have used Cornaro as a prototype and have surveyed his thought and his influence. We cannot consider in detail the very extensive literature devoted to the prolongation of life by means of hygiene. Just how numerous these treatises are, may be seen in the Shock bibliographies in the sections devoted to publications before 1900 [43]; an analysis of this material would make an interesting monograph. Here, however, attention will be restricted to a few representative works. One important regimen not included is that of Francis Bacon; it is too complex and too closely linked with his plans for experimental medicine to be classified as prolongevity hygiene, as here defined, and, therefore, will be considered in the next chapter.

Cornaro found an articulate disciple in Leonard Lessius, a Belgian Jesuit who stressed religious aspects of the temperate life. In Lessius' *Hygiasticon*, published in 1613, every one of Cornaro's theses finds an echo: like Cornaro, the Belgian scholar claimed that his life

was despaired of by the physicians until he adopted the sober life; he praised moderation especially in diet; he asserted that simple reforms in one's way of life will free one from virtually all disease and will insure a happy, healthy old age, an increase in longevity and an easy "natural" death. [44] Lessius called up the example of the "Holy-Men and Sage Philosophers of old" whose abstemious conduct gained them a long and useful life, and, like most of the hygienists, he had a special feeling for the simple peasants and artisans "who contentedly live on plain country fare, with temperance and due labor." [45] In the writings of the Jesuit thêre is less of the sunshine and exuberance of the Renaissance and more of the rigid discipline and self-denial of the Counter-Reformation. Yet, like Cornaro, he hoped to attain the best of both worlds, and his thoughts represent a curious mixture of earthly and heavenly aspirations:

For what can a Christian more desire, than after old age to enjoy his mind sound and healthful; cheerful, expedite, and vigorous to all the employments and functions thereof? For besides that it is very pleasant in its own nature, it carries along with it a very great spiritual advantage. For from long experience of fore-past age the vanity and emptiness of the world is the better discerned and becomes daily the more insipid. [46]

Such were the incongruous motives for the cleric's earnest endeavor to "preserve a sound mind in a sound body, and to add length of days to the short span of human life." [47]

For a more secular point of view, we may turn to Sir William Temple's essay, "Of Health and Long Life." [48] The seventeenth-century diplomat and *litterateur* was himself "too much the libertine" to value longevity at the price of a sober regimen; however, with the "intention of some public good," he brought together his observations on the subject, and they feature several of the typical notions of prolongevity hygiene. For one thing, there is the credulity about the life span: the natives of Brazil and the Brahmans of India are reported to live two to three hundred years, while the Hebrew patriarchs lived still longer; the explanation for this must be their natural and simple way of life. [49] The English essayist added with some pride that his own land had produced some cases of remarkable longevity even in modern times: [50] the most preeminent was "old Parr" who lived to nearly 153 "and might have, as was thought, gone further, if the change of country air and diet for that of the town had not carried him off." Then there was the Countess of Desmond who, though hounded by poverty,

[42] William Harvey, "The Anatomical Examination of the Body of Thomas Parr," in *The Works of William Harvey*, Robert Willis, transl. (London, 1847), pp. 587–592.
[43] Shock, *op. cit.* (see fn. 1).

[44] Lessius, *op. cit.* (see fn. 2).
[45] *Ibid.*, pp. 6, 40.
[46] *Ibid.*, p. 108.
[47] *Ibid.*, p. 109.
[48] William Temple, "Of Health and Long Life," in *The Works of Sir William Temple* (London, 1770) 3: pp. 266–303.
[49] *Ibid.*, pp. 271–272.
[50] *Ibid.*, pp. 275–278.

lived above 140. Temple asserted that he himself had met a beggar whose scant diet had brought him to the age of 124. The evidence indicated that the recipe for longevity was the temperate life:

... all the ... recites or observations, either of long-lived races or persons ... make it easy to conclude, that health and long life are usually blessings of the poor, not of the rich, and the fruits of temperance, rather than of luxury and excess.[51]

The greatest exponent of prolongevity hygiene, next to Cornaro, was the illustrious German physician Christopher Hufeland, who set the human life span at two hundred years. A member of the Weimar group, Hufeland was a friend of Goethe, Schiller, and Herder, while in medical circles he was known for introducing into Germany Jenner's new method for smallpox vaccination.[52] In his *Art of Prolonging Life* (later titled *Makrobiotik*), published in 1796, Hufeland saw impressive possibilities for improving longevity:

With regard to ... the absolute duration of human life, there is nothing to prevent us from giving it the utmost extent to which, according to experience, it is possible for it to attain. ... Now, experience incontestably tells us, that a man still may attain to the age of 150 or 160 years; and what is of the greatest importance is, that the instance of Thomas Parr, whose body was opened in his 152d year, proves that even at this age, the state of the bowels may be so perfect and sound that one might certainly live some time longer.[53]

Hufeland next cited the renowned physiologist Albrecht von Haller, who had collected statistics on unusual longevity: there were more than a thousand cases past the century mark, sixty above 110, twenty-nine above 120, fifteen over 130, six had surpassed 140, and the most long-lived of all, Henry Jenkins, was said to have reached 169.[54] Both Haller and Hufeland concluded that man could reach the age of 200, for, in addition to the above case histories, one might reason from comparative biology as follows: an animal, as a rule, lives eight times as long as its period of growth; man "in a natural state" requires 25 years to reach physical maturity; therefore, the human life span must be 8 × 25, or 200 years.[55] To give the argument a touch of Biblical authority, it was assumed that in very ancient times the year consisted of only about three months; thus, the 969 years of Methuselah would be reduced to the vicinity of 200.[56]

Hufeland had nothing but scorn for alchemy and the theories of Paracelsus, but he had a glowing admiration for Cornaro and his hypothesis that life may be lengthened by temperance.[57] The body, wrote the German physician, is born with a certain quantity of "vital power" which may be used up either quickly or slowly, depending on one's way of life.[58] To prolong life, it is necessary that this vital power be conserved; one must live *extensively* rather than *intensively*. Hufeland's code of hygiene was much more comprehensive than Cornaro's, ranging over such diverse topics as child care, the problem of suicide, and the way to recognize and evade a mad dog.[59] The *leitmotif* of the work, however, was similar to Cornaro's: moderation in all things, especially in diet.[60] As usual, the hygienic elite is made up of simple, working people in a rural environment:

The most extraordinary instances of longevity are to be found, however, only among those classes of mankind who, amidst bodily labor, and in the open air, lead a simple life agreeable to nature, such as farmers, gardeners, hunters, soldiers and sailors. In these situations man still attains to the age of 140, and even 150.[61]

The suppositions of prolongevity hygiene persisted far into the nineteenth century; a noteworthy illustration of this is William Sweetser's *Human Life*, published in 1867.[62] A professor of medicine at the University of Vermont, and later at Bowdoin, Sweetser is remembered for coining the term "mental hygiene."[63] In his work on prolongevity, there appear all the famous cases of unusual longevity: Henry Jenkins, Thomas Parr, etc., and to these are added some American contributions, the most recent being Joseph Crele "of Wisconsin" who died in 1866 at the age of 141.[64] Sweetser's conclusion is that,

Admitting now that some of the instances of extraordinary longevity which have been introduced, are overstated, and others not fully attested, yet with such allowance, there will remain enough of well authenticated examples to show that human existence has endured for more than a century and a half.[65]

As expected, one of the chief means proposed for attaining such a duration of life was temperance[66]; however, the New England physician also was influenced by developments outside the Cornaro tradition: he was a Darwinist and a staunch believer in the idea of progress; consequently, his hopes for prolongevity

[51] *Ibid.*, p. 278.
[52] Zeman, *op. cit.* (see fn. 1) **12** (1945): p. 949 and Grmek, *op. cit.* (see fn. 1), pp. 67–68.
[53] Christopher William Hufeland, *The Art of Prolonging Life* (2 v., London, 1797) **1**: pp. 175–176.
[54] *Ibid.*, pp. 141–142, 179.
[55] *Ibid.*, pp. 176–177.
[56] *Ibid.*, pp. 121–122.
[57] *Ibid.*, pp. 10–14, 21–25. Hufeland warned, however, that Cornaro's own regimen was too severe for most patients.
[58] *Ibid.*, pp. 62–65, 69–73.
[59] *Ibid.* **2**: *passim*.
[60] *Ibid.* **1**: p. 167.
[61] *Ibid.*, p. 141.
[62] William Sweetser, *Human Life: Considered in its Present Condition and Future Developments, Especially with Reference to its Duration* (New York, 1867).
[63] Howard A. Kelly and Walter L. Burrage, *Dictionary of American Medical Biography* (New York and London, 1928), p. 1182 and Arturo Castiglioni, *A History of Medicine*, E. B. Krumbhaar, transl. (New York, 1947), p. 1102.
[64] Sweetser, *op. cit.* (see fn. 62), pp. 164–180.
[65] *Ibid.*, pp. 179–180.
[66] *Ibid.*, pp. 217–238.

were centered, for the most part, on future advances in medical science.[67] Meanwhile, on a more popular level, the Cornaro theme continued in full force; for example, D. H. Jacques' *Physical Perfection,* published in 1859, included a chapter on "The Secret of Longevity."[68] The secret, of course, is moderation in all things; for, "the energy of life is in inverse ratio with its duration."[69] Jacques also mentions ten "well-authenticated" instances of persons in modern times living beyond 150. The hero of the essay is Cornaro, who demonstrated "the extent to which one's health and longevity are in his own hands."[70]

CONCLUSION

By the last quarter of the nineteenth century, the main tenets of prolongevity hygiene had become seriously challenged, largely because of the rise of bacteriology and vital statistics. Already during the eighteenth century, the "benevolent despots" of Europe had begun to accept the idea that health is a responsibility of the state rather than of the individual; this trend was continued by the reforms of the French Revolution.[71] In the nineteenth century, the problems of industrialization and urbanization stimulated the Sanitation Movement with a further extension of *social* hygiene.[72] The heaviest blows to traditional, personal hygiene came with the development of antisepsis, anesthesia, and bacteriology; medicine now had effective weapons against disease: vaccines, antitoxins, precision surgery, and the complex techniques of epidemiology. In contrast with this powerful arsenal of organized medicine and public health, it could be maintained no longer with Cornaro that "a man can have no better doctor than himself."[73]

At the same time, the belief in super-centenarians was eroded by the combined methods of statistical analysis and historical criticism. The turning point was the publication in 1873 of William J. Thoms' *Human Longevity, its Facts and its Fictions.*[74] Thoms, a librarian at the House of Lords, was, in his spare time, an antiquarian and is noted for introducing the word "folklore."[75] In his work on longevity, he blamed physicians for their gullibility and turned instead to the life insurance statisticians for reliable evidence on the duration of life.[76] Next he laid down the requirements which must be met before a case of extraordinary longevity could be accepted as valid.[77] He especially took issue with the idea that poor inhabitants of rural areas were the most long-lived, pointing out that these were the very localities in which records were most inadequate.[78] A chapter was devoted to disproving each of the renowned English cases of long life: Henry Jenkins, Thomas Parr, and the Countess of Desmond.[79] These activities brought Thoms into bitter controversy, for Jenkins had been honored with an expensive monument by his fellow Yorkshiremen, while Parr had been interred in Westminster Abbey.[80]

If in doubting the 169 years of Henry Jenkins, I have been guilty of an act of daring scepticism; what can be said in extenuation of my still greater audacity in doubting the 152 years of Thomas Parr? . . . There is no doubt that Thomas Parr was a very old man, an exceptionally old man; probably a hundred.[81]

With his spirited, rather sarcastic arguments, Thoms destroyed one of the chief pillars of prolongevity hygiene.[82] If the life span was limited to one hundred, as he asserted, then the hope of greatly extending the length of life no longer could be focused on simply conserving the body's vital powers. It appeared that God and Nature had not been so generous in allotting years to man, and if he desired a greater longevity, he would have to achieve some significant breakthrough in science and medicine.

VIII. THE *PHILOSOPHES*

The rapid progress *true* science now makes, occasions my regretting sometimes that I was born so soon. It is impossible to imagine the height to which may be carried, in a thousand years, the power of man over matter. We may perhaps learn to deprive large masses of their gravity, and give them absolute levity, for the sake of easy transport. Agriculture may diminish its labor and double its produce; all diseases may by sure means be prevented or cured, not excepting even that of old age, and our lives lengthened at pleasure even beyond the antediluvian standard.

Benjamin Franklin, Letter to Priestley, 1780.[1]

DEATH AND PROGRESS

The idea of progress thoroughly revolutionized men's views about the prolongation of life. With the possible exception of Renaissance hygiene, all the major schools of prolongevitism—folklore, Taoism, alchemy—

[67] *Ibid.,* pp. 275–279.

[68] Daniel Harrison Jacques, *Physical Perfection: or, the Philosophy of Human Beauty; Showing how to Acquire and Retain Bodily Symmetry, Health and Vigor, Secure Long Life, and Avoid the Infirmities and Deformities of Age* (New York, 1859), pp. 207–220.

[69] *Ibid.,* p. 212.

[70] *Ibid.,* p. 220.

[71] George Rosen, *A History of Public Health* (New York, 1958), pp. 161–170.

[72] *Ibid.,* pp. 192 ff.

[73] *Cf.* Richard H. Shryock, *The Development of Modern Medicine* (Philadelphia, 1936), chap. 13: "Public Confidence Lost" and 16: "Public Confidence Regained."

[74] William J. Thoms, *Human Longevity, its Facts and its Fictions* (London, 1873).

[75] Zeman, *op. cit.* (see fn. 1) 17 (1950): pp. 56–58.

[76] Thoms, *op. cit.* (see fn. 74), pp. 7–13, 27–30.

[77] *Ibid.,* pp. 31–66.

[78] *Ibid.,* pp. 18–30.

[79] *Ibid.,* pp. 67–104.

[80] On Jenkins' monument, see *ibid.,* pp. 78–79.

[81] *Ibid.,* p. 85.

[82] Thoms' work aroused the British Medical Association to set up committees to collect accurate statistics on disease and old age; Zeman, *op. cit.* (see fn. 1) 17 (1950): pp. 57–58.

[1] Benjamin Franklin, *Works,* John Bigelow, ed. (New York, 1904) 8: pp. 174–175.

had been founded on primitivism, the belief that pro-longevity already had been achieved in the past. The advent of the idea of progress presented a completely different vision to the human imagination: prolongevity as a goal to be attained in the future. The idea of progress may be defined, with Bury, as the belief "that civilization has moved, is moving, and will move in a desirable direction." [2] If one believed in progress and thought the prolongation of life to be desirable, then it followed that one of the attainable goals of humanity must be increased longevity.

Thus, prolongevitism evolved as a corollary of the idea of progress. No longer was it necessary for pro-ponents of prolongevitism to attempt shamefaced ex-planations of the apparent inability of adepts to lengthen their own lives; one merely could remark, with Franklin, that the present generation was "born too soon." There was no longer need for the dogmatic cult of esoteric "secrets" alleged to have been handed down from the sages of old; the wisdom of the past lost its hegemony, and one could speak boldly of aiming *beyond* the ante-diluvian standard. The suspicious and secretive factions of initiates gave way to a *"true* science," in which re-search was carried on in a cooperative way, while errors were rooted out in open debate.

With the idea of progress, prolongevitism for the first time made its way to the center of the stage in Western civilization. The process of recognition had begun with Latin alchemy, the first significant system of prolongevitism in the West. A further foothold was marked by Renaissance hygiene. But the turning-point came in the eighteenth century, when the belief in progress undermined most of the traditional strong-points of apologism.[3] The Epicurean view that there was nothing new under the sun, that lengthened life would be a wearying round of the same experiences, now was replaced by the expectation of change and improvement. The Stoic view of man as a fragile and pathetic creature was superseded by hopes for increas-ing human power over natural forces. In the light of the potentialities of modern science, the cautious objec-tives of the Galen-Avicenna type of medicine seemed pusillanimous. And the traditional Christian preference for other-worldly aspirations was countered by a new dream which envisioned a veritable heaven on earth.

During the nineteenth century, the idea of progress had become so widespread that it seemed almost a self-evident principle. It remained for scholarly studies, most notably that of Bury, to trace the evolution of the concept and to demonstrate that its ascendancy had oc-curred only during the modern era.[4] In antiquity, the

two main theories of history were those of regression and cycles; the regression theory we have become familiar with, because its variant, primitivism, was identified with early systems of prolongevity. The cyclical theory, of course, pictured society following a path of alternat-ing ups and down without any overall headway. There were, along with these dominant trends, a few glimmer-ings of progressist thought. One of these centered on the prospect of a return of the Age of Gold: both the Hebrews and the early Christians harbored millennial hopes of a New Jerusalem; and, in a more secular vein, Vergil, in the glow of the Augustan principate, wrote his famous passage suggesting an imminent rebirth of hu-manity.[5] The other type of early speculation about progress was related to advances expected in science and the mechanical arts. The model expression of this senti-ment was that of Seneca in his remarks on the dis-coveries reserved for future ages when learned men will "clear up problems which are now obscure" and "marvel at our ignorance of causes so clear to them." [6] The same thought was repeated by al-Razi, amplified by Jabir and further elaborated on by Roger Bacon.[7] But, according to Bury, the clear enunciation of the idea of progress could not occur until the groundwork had been prepared by the seventeenth-century philosophers Des-cartes and Francis Bacon, both of whom, it may be noted, were keenly concerned with the prolongation of life.

The first full-bodied expressions of faith in progress appeared during the eighteenth century. Interestingly enough, they usually reflect the same two beliefs which had stimulated the earliest anticipations of the possibility of human advance: the return of the golden age (millen-nialism) and the growth of science and the arts. These were the two inspirations, for example, for Richard Price's *Evidence for a Future Period of Improvement*.[8] Price began by calling to witness the prophetic state-ments of Daniel, Isaiah, and Paul in support of his con-tention that

Hitherto the kingdom of the Messiah has been in its in-fancy. The most glorious period of it is yet future. . . . The light it has hitherto produced has been like the dawn

---

[2] J. B. Bury, *The Idea of Progress* (New York, 1932), p. 2.

[3] On apologism, see earlier, chap. II.

[4] Bury, *op. cit.* (see fn. 2). Other standard works on the subject are Jules Delvaille, *Essai sur l'histoire de l'idée de progrès, jusqu'à la fin du XVIIIᵉ siècle*, Collection historique des grands philosophes (Paris, 1910); Carl L. Becker, *The Heavenly City of the Eighteenth-Century Philosophers* (New

Haven, 1932); R. V. Sampson, *Progress in the Age of Rea-son: the Seventeenth Century to the Present Day* (Cambridge, Mass., 1956); Frederick J. Teggart and George H. Hildebrand, eds., *The Idea of Progress: A Collection of Readings* (Berke-ley and Los Angeles, 1949). On the eighteenth-century belief in progress, see also Crane Brinton, *Ideas and Men* (2nd ed., Englewood Cliffs, N. J., 1963), pp. 294–318, and *A History of Western Morals* (New York, 1959), pp. 293–328; and Kingsley Martin, *French Liberal Thought in the Eighteenth Century* (3rd ed., London, 1962 and New York, 1963), pp. 277–305.

[5] On hopes for a return of the Age of Gold, see earlier, chap. III, section on the antediluvian theme.

[6] Bury, *op. cit.* (see fn. 2), pp. 13–15.

[7] See earlier, chap. VI.

[8] Richard Price, *The Evidence for a Future Period of Im-provement in the State of Mankind, with the Means and Duty of Promoting It* (London, 1787).

of the morning. It will hereafter produce a bright day over the whole earth.[9]

Having sounded revelation, the English dissenter turned to the testimony of reason and recalled how the labors of the ancients had prepared the way for the prodigies of recent times, Bacon, Boyle, and Newton.[10]

One generation thus improved communicates improvement to the next, and that to the next, till at last a progress in improvement may take place rapid and irresistible, which may issue in the happiest state of things that can exist on this earth.[11]

It was but a step from this to meliorism, the belief that human action can improve the world:

There is great encouragement in this consideration. It shows us that the greatest good may arise from the slightest degree of real improvement, which we can produce by our exertions; and it should, therefore, quicken our zeal in all such exertions.[12]

The ease with which these ideas of progress, meliorism, and the perfectability of man, blended with prolongevity is indicated by the well-known statement of Price's friend, Joseph Priestley:

. . . and knowledge, as Lord Bacon observes, being power, the human powers will, in fact, be enlarged; nature, including both its materials, and its laws, will be more at our command; men will make their situation in this world abundantly more easy and comfortable; they will probably prolong their existence in it. . . .[13]

The most fruitful interpretation, for our purposes, of the eighteenth-century idea of progress is the now nearly classical work of Carl Becker.[14] According to Becker, it is incorrect to class together ancient and medieval ideas about the meaning of history, even though both were similar in lacking the idea of progress; actually, there was a tremendous difference between the ancient and the medieval outlook. The Greeks and Romans were basically without much hope in regard to the future of society. The medieval Christian, on the contrary, looked forward to the salvation of all mankind; indeed, this was the purpose of history. The Christian may have been pessimistic and scornful concerning the things of this world, but he believed that, by means of divine intervention, all would be made right in the great resurrection and judgment at the end of the historical process. To medieval Christendom, the world was a great stage on which was acted out the intense and meaningful drama of salvation.

The great ideas of the eighteenth-century Enlightenment, according to Becker, were based on a secularization of the medieval Christian drama of salvation, i.e., its transformation into the idea of progress towards a heaven on earth.[15] The modern temper, he wrote, owes more to the culture of medieval times than to that of the Greeks and Romans. The philosophe of the eighteenth century may have ridiculed traditional religion, but he himself represented the beginnings of a new religion—a religion of progress. It is incorrect, therefore, to speak of an age of reason superseding an age of faith. Where medieval man put his faith in supernatural methods, the philosophe centered his faith on man and nature. While Christianity was other-worldly, the philosophes were concerned with this world. But both movements were based on faith, and both were motivated by the devout desire to save mankind. The truly religious nature of the Enlightenment was revealed, Becker wrote, when the Jacobins gained power in revolutionary France and put into effect a pious system of secular ceremonials, feast days, and creeds.[16]

For us, the most intriguing part of Becker's thesis is his last chapter, "The Uses of Posterity," in which he dealt with the problem of death. There he pointed out that, in place of the Christian promise of immortality, the philosophes substituted the hope that virtuous men might live forever in the memory of future generations. While Christians had sought salvation from death by means of supernatural resurrection and immortality, the philosophes, according to Becker, tried to achieve a similar goal by founding a cult of heroes who had benefited humanity. Grateful men of the future would judge which of their ancestors were most worthy of "resurrection," and the names of the chosen would be entered in the pantheon of fame. Becker suggested that the vision of such a future apotheosis might sustain the virtuous philosophe in the same way that a good Christian was enheartened by thoughts of the resurrection and judgment to come, and, in this regard, Becker quoted Diderot's remark, "Posterity is for the philosopher what the other world is to the man of religion."

"The Uses of Posterity" is so important, because it brings to our attention the contradiction between death and progress; but, unfortunately, Becker touches on this problem only lightly and indirectly. The cult of the

---

[9] Ibid., p. 4, see also pp. 6–11.
[10] Ibid., pp. 14–16, 21.
[11] Ibid., p. 36.
[12] Ibid., p. 35.
[13] Joseph Priestley, An Essay on the First Principles of Government (2nd ed., London, 1771), p. 4.
[14] Becker, op. cit. (see fn. 4). There are many criticisms, most of them peripheral, in Raymond O. Rockwood, ed., Carl Becker's Heavenly City Revisited (Ithaca, N. Y., 1958). Peter Gay attacks Becker in a spirited essay reprinted in his The Party of Humanity: Essays in the French Enlightenment (New York, 1964), pp. 188–210. Much can be learned about Becker's point of view by reading his early and brilliant essay "Kansas" (1910), reprinted in his Everyman His Own Historian (New York, 1935), pp. 1–28. See also the excellent work by Burleigh Taylor Wilkins, Carl Becker: A Biographical Study in American Intellectual History (Cambridge, Mass., 1961).

[15] Becker, op. cit. (see fn. 4), pp. 29 ff.
[16] Ibid., pp. 155 ff. Cf. Crane Brinton, The Jacobins: an Essay in the New History (New York, 1930 and 1961), especially chap. 6, "Ritual," and chap. 7, "Faith." The interpretation of the French Revolution in terms of "secular religion" has been criticized by Peter Gay and defended by Crane Brinton in the Amer. Historical Review 66 (1961): pp. 664–681; Brinton cites Condorcet's radical prolongevitism as a form of natural salvation or secular eschatology (p. 680).

hero by no means can be considered a complete secular substitute for the far-reaching medieval scheme of supernatural salvation. Medieval Christianity provided an historical outlook which not only saw meaning and purpose in history but included in that dramatic denouement the salvation of mankind from its great enemy, death. In the Christian system, each and every believer could look forward to an actual resurrection from the grave. Compared to that, how puny must have seemed the Enlightenment cult of the hero, by which a select few would live on as disembodied memories in the consciousness of some future generation. Such an ethereal type of immortality could not prove entirely satisfactory to a pattern of thought which focused its attention on achieving on this earth a real flesh-and-blood counterpart of heaven.

While there may have been some *philosophes* sentimental enough to be gratified completely by thoughts of posthumous fame, there always were others who pushed onward, seeking a more tangible form of victory over death. As soon as the idea of progress began to take hold, philosophers like Bacon and Descartes were grappling with the problem of the prolongation of life. No sooner did man's confidence in supernatural salvation begin to weaken, than the released energies began to be diverted into an intensified effort to lengthen life on this earth. Of course, such a radical intellectual transformation could not be carried out in a completely conscious and direct manner; Bacon and Descartes were torn between tradition and innovation, between faith in divine power and faith in the power of man. Only gradually were even the most advanced thinkers able to formulate and express a bold and optimistic attitude towards death. About the middle of the eighteenth century, Priestley, as we have seen, spoke of progress bringing about prolongevity, while Franklin in 1780 ventured the prediction that longevity might reach beyond a thousand years. But not till Godwin and Condorcet, near the end of the century, do we see the Enlightenment faith being carried towards its logical conclusion with the assertion that mankind should be able to attain immortality on earth.

THE SEVENTEENTH CENTURY

DESCARTES [17]

Although it is customary to contrast Descartes with Bacon, there is at least one striking similarity: both aimed for useful knowledge, both believed science could enable man to ameliorate his situation in this world.[18] To be sure, in methodology they were very different; Bacon favored an empirical, qualitative, rather piecemeal approach, while Descartes was more theoretical, mathematical, and speculative. But the goal was the same: practical information to allow the human conquest of nature. In Descartes, this is seen in his *Discourse on the Method,* the work in which his enthusiasm for science and meliorism is most clearly revealed; indeed, the original title was the grandiose, *Project for a Universal Science Able to Raise our Nature to its Highest Degree of Perfection.*[19] The author relates how his desire for clear, certain, and useful knowledge led him to abandon schools and books and venture into the world of action.[20] In 1617 he joined the forces of Maurice of Nassau, a master of military engineering and applied mathematics; the Netherlands at the time was the scene of extraordinary material improvement and scientific advance.[21]

These experiences of Descartes are reflected in the *Discourse,* where he speaks of "the law by which we are bound to promote, as far as in us lies, the general good of mankind" and continues,

. . . I perceived it to be possible to arrive at knowledge highly useful in life; and in room of the speculative philosophy usually taught in the schools, to discover a practical, by means of which, knowing the force and action of fire, water, air, the stars, the heavens, and all the other bodies that surround us, as distinctly as we know the various crafts of our artisans, we might also apply them in the same way to all the uses to which they are adapted, and thus render ourselves the lords and possessors of nature.[22]

As his biographer Adam noted, Descartes blended the logic of scholasticism with the Faustian dreams of medieval artisans and alchemists.[23]

In Descartes' scheme of applied science, medicine held the chief position; he compared philosophy to a tree with three fruitbearing branches: mechanics, medicine, and ethics, and ethics he believed to be founded on medicine.[24] Perhaps because of his sickly childhood, he affirmed health to be the greatest benefit in life.

And this [the conquest of nature] is a result to be desired, not only in order to the invention of an infinity of arts, by which we might be enabled to enjoy without any trouble the fruits of the earth, and all its comforts, but also and

[17] The classic biography of Descartes is that of Adrien Baillet, *La Vie de Descartes* (2 v., Paris, 1691). The best modern one is Charles Adam, *Vie et œuvres de Descartes: étude historique* (Paris, 1910); hereafter referred to as "Adam, *Vie.*" Also useful are Elizabeth S. Haldane, *Descartes: his Life and Times* (London, 1905) and J. P. Mahaffy, *Descartes,* Philosophical Classics for English Readers (Edinburgh and London, 1902). The definitive edition of his works is that of Charles Adam and Paul Tannery (11 v., Paris, 1897–1909); hereafter referred to as "Descartes, *Œuvres.*"

[18] On seventeenth-century French interest in applied science, see Harcourt Brown, "The Utilitarian Motive in the Age of Descartes," *Annals of Science* 1 (1936): pp. 182–192.

[19] Adam, *Vie,* p. 228.

[20] René Descartes, *Discourse on the Method of Rightly Conducting the Reason, and Seeking Truth in the Sciences* in John Veitch, transl., *A Discourse on Method, etc.,* Everyman's Library (London, Toronto and New York, 1912), pp. 5–9; this treatise is hereafter referred to as "Descartes, *Discourse.*"

[21] Haldane, *op. cit.* (see fn. 17), pp. 41–44.

[22] Descartes, *Discourse,* p. 49.

[23] Adam, *Vie,* pp. 227–230.

[24] Descartes, *Œuvres* 9, 2, p. 14 and *Discourse,* p. 49.

especially for the preservation of health, which is without doubt, of all the blessings of this life, the first and fundamental one.[25]

In concluding the *Discourse,* Descartes vowed to further the advance of medicine:

. . . I have resolved to devote what time I may still have to live to no other occupation than that of endeavoring to acquire some knowledge of Nature, which shall be of such a kind as to enable us therefrom to deduce rules in medicine of greater certainty than those at present in use.[26]

The philosopher, of course, did not fulfill this pledge to give up his other interests; it is true, however, that he devoted a great part of his time to medical studies and to the company of physicians.[27] He was especially proficient at anatomical dissection and also did a little clinical work and elaborated some hypotheses on pathology and therapy. And his *Treatise on Man* was a landmark in the history of physiology.[28]

A primary motivation for Descartes' medical investigations was his desire for prolonged life. In the *Discourse,* he spoke hopefully of a possible cure for senescence:

. . . all at present known in it [medicine] is almost nothing in comparison of what remains to be discovered . . . we could free ourselves from an infinity of maladies of body as well as of mind, and perhaps also even from the debility of age, if we had sufficiently ample knowledge of their causes, and of all the remedies provided for us by nature.[29]

Also, in the preface to his *Description of the Human Body,* he stated that, regarding medicine,

. . . I believe it may be possible to find many very sound precepts for the cure of diseases and for their prevention and also even for the retardation of aging. . . .[30]

Feeling he had discovered a sure path for advancing science and philosophy, Descartes was highly desirous to live long enough to see the bountiful results of his

---

[25] Descartes, *Discourse,* p. 49. *Cf.* his statement in a letter of October, 1645: "The conservation of health has been at all times the principal goal of my studies . . ."; Descartes, *Œuvres* 4: p. 329.

[26] Descartes, *Discourse,* p. 61.

[27] Haldane, *op. cit.* (see fn. 17), pp. 126–127; Smith, *op. cit.* (see below, fn. 28), pp. 341–342; and Berthier, *op. cit.* (see below, fn. 28) 2: pp. 43–46. For a thorough account of Descartes' medical work, see H. Dreyfus-Le Foyer, "Les Conceptions médicales de Descartes," *Revue de métaphysique et de morale* 44 (1937): pp. 237–286.

[28] *Traité de l'homme* in Descartes, *Œuvres* 11: pp. 118–215. On Descartes' contribution to physiology, see the introductory accounts by Charles Singer, *A History of Biology* (rev. ed., New York, 1950), pp. 354–357; Michael Foster, *Lectures on the History of Physiology During the Sixteenth, Seventeenth and Eighteenth Centuries* (Cambridge, 1901), pp. 57–62, 260–269; and Norman Kemp Smith, *New Studies in the Philosophy of Descartes: Descartes as Pioneer* (London, 1952), pp. 124–137. A detailed study is Auguste Georges Berthier, "Le Mécanisme cartésien et la physiologie au XVIIᵉ siècle," *Isis* 2 (1914): pp. 37–89, and 3 (1920): pp. 21–58.

[29] Descartes, *Discourse,* p. 50.

[30] Descartes, *Œuvres* 11: pp. 223–224.

labor; he was intensely aware that art is long and life is short, and, consequently, he frequently expressed concern about health and longevity. In the *Discourse,* for example, he spoke of his great "expectations of the future," but, at the same time, he felt uneasy about the "brief duration of my life." [31] Similarly, he expressed confidence that one employing his methodology must inevitably reach the end desired *unless* hindered "by the shortness of life." [32] Thus, with the appearance of the idea of progress, there arises a feeling that it is desirable to prolong life; a yearning which makes an interesting contrast to the Epicurean concept of the "fullness of pleasure," according to which prolongevity is not desirable, because there is never anything new under the sun.[33]

Descartes was very circumspect regarding opinions which might bring him into conflict with the Church, and he did not publish any detailed views on prolongevity; indeed, even his treatise on physiology, which was to have accompanied the *Discourse,* was voluntarily suppressed and did not appear until after his death.[34] His correspondence is not much more helpful, as he intended it for publication, and, therefore, maintained in it a good bit of self-restraint.[35] There is, however, one occasion when his zeal escaped the usual controls; in a letter to Constantyn Huygens, father of the great scientist, he wrote,

. . . I now will satisfy you on the last point raised in your letter, by telling you with what I am occupying myself. I never took so much care to conserve myself as I do now, and, though I had thought formerly that death could not rob me of more than thirty or forty years, henceforth it cannot surprise me without depriving me of the hope of more than a century: since it seems to me evident that if we guard ourselves from certain errors which we customarily commit in our way of life, we will be able without other inventions to achieve an old age much longer and happier than now; but because I need much time and experience to examine all that pertains to this subject, I am working now on an abridgment of medicine, which is drawn in part from books and partly from reasoning, and which I hope will serve to obtain for me some delay of nature and so be able afterwards to better pursue my aim.[36]

The ambiguous wording in this passage makes it impossible to determine whether Descartes meant to say that he hoped to live to more than a hundred, or that he expected a hundred years in addition to his present age; as he was forty-two at the time, the latter interpretation would indicate that he sought to reach a hundred forty or a hundred fifty.

---

[31] Descartes, *Discourse,* p. 4.

[32] *Ibid.,* p. 50.

[33] See earlier, chap. II, section on philosophy.

[34] Singer, *op. cit.* (see fn. 28), p. 354.

[35] Mahaffy, *op. cit.* (see fn. 17), p. 5.

[36] January 25, 1638; Descartes, *Œuvres* 1: p. 507. On Huygens' reply asking for more information, see Leon Roth, ed., *Correspondence of Descartes and Constantyn Huygens: 1635–1647* (Oxford, 1926), p. 80.

Other information concerning Descartes' interest in prolongevity comes from indirect sources; St. Evremond, for example, gave his biographer an account of a visit of Sir Kenelm Digby to the great philosopher. After an exchange of rather highflown compliments,

... Sir Kenelm said to this Philosopher, "That our speculative discoveries were indeed pretty and agreeable, but that after all they were too uncertain and unprofitable to take up a man's whole thoughts: that life was almost too short to attain to the right knowledge of necessary things, and that it would be much more worthy of him, who so well understood the frame of the human body, to study ways and means to prolong it, than to apply himself to bare speculations of philosophy." M. Des Cartes assured him, that he had already considered that matter; and that to render a man immortal, was what he would not venture to promise, but that he was very sure it was possible to lengthen out his life to the period of the Patriarchs.[37]

St. Evremond is said to have added that Descartes' hopes for the prolongation of life were well known in Holland, and that he himself had confirmed the stories by consulting friends of the late philosopher.

Further data regarding prolongevity concern Descartes' disciple the Abbé Picot, who, according to Baillet, adopted a temperate diet, in the belief that this was one of the means by which the philosopher would extend the life span to four or five hundred years.[38] The same abbé is said to have been deeply shocked and incredulous at the news of Descartes' death at the age of only fifty-four; he insisted that some remarkably violent cause must have been involved, for he had fully expected the sage to attain the means of reaching the age of five hundred.[39] Moreover, during Descartes' last months, in Sweden, he is reported to have spoken hopefully of lengthening life to an extraordinary degree, and Queen Christina had the impression that he sought to live forever.[40]

All this gives only one side of the picture, for Descartes was torn by inner conflicts regarding his rationalism, utilitarianism, and prolongevitism. The philosopher's waverings on the question of rationalism are well known; perhaps because of gratitude to his early educators, the Jesuits, and also because of his alarm at the condemnation of Galileo, Descartes took great pains to avoid challenging the Faith.[41] The deep emotional roots of this conflict were indicated by the terrifying dream of 1619 in which he was caught up by a fierce wind which swept him first towards and then away from a church; drenched in perspiration, he awoke with

the passage in mind, "What path shall I follow in life?"[42]

As a result of this sort of irresolution, his system of thought is rent by a sharp dualism. In the *Discourse,* he swears to follow unswervingly the dictates of reason, and yet, at the same time, he vows an almost unconditional loyalty to the customs of his country and the precepts of his religion.[43] He waxes enthusiastic, in the most modern manner, over the possibilities of science for remaking the world, and then avows in the Stoic tradition that the mission of ethics is to teach men to submit to the world as it is.[44] In one letter, as we have seen, he set forth his desire to prolong life, yet in another he wrote, ". . . in place of finding the means to conserve life, I have found another, much easier and more certain, that of losing the fear of death."[45] It is revealing of the pressures under which he worked, that his disciples had to defend him against accusations of impiety based on the charge that he endeavored to achieve prolongevity.[46]

While Descartes did not leave any explicit account of how he hoped to attain prolongevity, one idea he seems to have tried was a regimen like that of Cornaro, or perhaps more elaborate, like the dietary techniques of the Taoists.[47] His optimism also stemmed from the belief that he himself had made two great contributions to physiology: the introduction of a clear and exact method of reasoning similar to the axioms of geometry and the initiation of a thorough-going mechanistic interpretation of the bodily functions. As seen in the *Discourse,* the philosopher felt that fundamental scientific advances would result from the application of geometrical reasoning.[48] More influential in the long run, however, was his conception of the body as a machine: man is like "a statue or machine of clay," and the activities of the organism are analogous to the working of mechanisms in which water, piped into the tubing under pressure, produces complex effects, as in water clocks, mills, and amusement-park displays.[49]

So long as vitalism held the field, physicians could not hope for a precise understanding of the workings of the body, but now all such phenomena were reduced to mechanical interrelationships.

The multitude and order of the nerves, veins, bones, and other parts of an animal, do not at all indicate that Nature is not adequate to form them, provided it is supposed

---

[37] P. Des Maizeaux, ed. and transl., *The Works of St. Evremond, with the Life of the Author by Des Maizeaux* (2nd ed., London, 1728) 1: pp. xli–xlii. On the antediluvian patriarchs, see earlier, chap. III.

[38] Baillet, *op. cit.* (see fn. 17) 2: p. 448.

[39] *Ibid.,* pp. 452–453; Baillet, however, denied Descartes had this intention.

[40] Adam, *Vie,* pp. 551–552, 581–582.

[41] On Descartes' "double life," see Haldane, *op. cit.* (see fn. 17), pp. 169–170; on how the Galileo episode tangled his system of thought, see Adam, *Vie,* pp. 165–179.

[42] A lively account of Descartes' dream (and part of its ideological background) is Jacques Maritain, *The Dream of Descartes, Together with some Other Essays,* Mabelle L. Andison, transl. (New York, 1944), pp. 11–29.

[43] Descartes, *Discourse,* pp. 19–23.

[44] *Ibid.,* pp. 49, 21–22.

[45] June 15, 1646; Descartes, *Œuvres* 4: p. 442.

[46] Adam, *Vie,* pp. 581–582.

[47] Descartes favored small but frequent meals of low-calorie foods such as fruit and "roots" but not meat; Baillet, *op. cit.* (see fn. 17) 2: p. 448.

[48] Descartes, *Discourse,* pp. 16–17.

[49] Descartes, *Œuvres* 11: pp. 120, 130–131.

that Nature acts in every case according to the precise laws of mechanics, and that God has imposed those laws on her. . . . I have found no thing whose particular formation I do not think myself able to explain by natural causes, just as I have explained in my *Meteors* that of a grain of salt, or of a small flake of snow.[50]

Here again, prolongevitism stimulated a fruitful development in biology and medicine. The alchemists' desire for long life, as we have seen, contributed to iatrochemistry, which later aided significantly the evolution of modern biochemistry and chemotherapy[51]; and Descartes, inspired also with the hope of increasing longevity, gave a strong impetus to iatrophysics, which in turn was an important element in the establishing of modern experimental physiology.

FRANCIS BACON [52]

There is no need to stress the meliorism of Francis Bacon; he is the very personification of the idea. To him, the purpose of the sciences is to increase human well-being by gaining a greater command over nature, and the true goal of research is "that human life be endowed with new discoveries and powers." [53] This meliorism was the guiding faith at "Solomon's House," the research center of Bacon's utopia, "New Atlantis."

The end of our foundation is the knowledge of causes, and secret motions of things; and the enlarging of the bounds of human empire, to the effecting of all things possible.[54]

Furthermore, Bacon felt that meliorism rebounded to the advantage of pure science itself:

. . . the practical results are not only the means to improve human well-being. They are also the guarantee of truth. There is a true rule in religion, that a man must show his faith by his works. The same rule holds good in natural philosophy. Science too must be known by its works. It is by the witness of works rather than by logic or even observation that the truth is revealed and established. It follows from this that the improvement of man's

lot and the improvement of man's mind are one and the same thing.[55]

And, like Descartes, Bacon felt that he had discovered a methodology which promised very extensive progress in the future.

There is therefore much ground for hoping that there are still laid up in the womb of nature many secrets of excellent use . . . by the method of which we are now treating they can be speedily and suddenly and simultaneously presented and anticipated.[56]

Prolongevity was a central concern in Bacon's meliorism; this view is expressed in his commentary on the myth of Prometheus.[57] In the account of Bacon, Prometheus gives fire to men, yet they complain to Zeus, and the ruler of the gods, in a benevolent mood, gives them, in addition, the boon of perpetual youth. But mankind improvidently allows a wily serpent to carry off the secret, whereby serpents, rather than men, have the power of restoring their youth (i.e., by the periodic shedding of skin).[58] Bacon's opinion was that this fable teaches that the divine powers desire men to be dissatisfied with the "defects of nature and art" and to strive for the highest degree of knowledge and power. In support of this interpretation, he observed that it was only after men had assumed a complaining and demanding attitude that the gods granted them the gift of eternal youth. The lesson is that,

. . . it seems to show that methods and medicines for the retardation of age and the prolongation of life were by the ancients not despaired of, but reckoned rather among those things which men once had and by sloth and negligence let slip, than among those which were wholly denied or never offered.[59]

This is typical of Bacon's middle position between primitivism and progressism; he was fond of citing the achievements of the ancients, but, at the same time, he often implied that they well might be overshadowed by the advances of the future.[60]

Bacon further explained his ideas on longevity in his *Advancement of Learning,* where he praised prolongevity as the "most noble" goal of medicine.

For if such a thing may be discovered, the business of medicine will no longer be confined to humble cures, nor will physicians be honoured only for necessity; but for a gift to men—of earthly gifts perhaps the greatest—of which, next to God, they may become the dispensers and administrators.[61]

[50] *Ibid.* 2: p. 525; translation by Aram Vartanian, *Diderot and Descartes: a Study of Scientific Naturalism in the Enlightenment,* History of Ideas Series 6 (Princeton, 1953), p. 247.
[51] See earlier, chap. VI, section on Latin alchemy.
[52] The standard biography is James Spedding, *An Account of the Life and Times of Francis Bacon* (2 v., Boston, 1878); one which accentuates his meliorism is Benjamin Farrington, *Francis Bacon: Philosopher of Industrial Science* (London, 1951). There is an interesting but unannotated survey of his medical work by Max Neuburger, "Lord Bacon's Relations to Medicine," *Medical Life* 33 (1926): pp. 149–169. The most satisfactory collection of his works is that of James Spedding, Robert Leslie Ellis and Douglas Denon Heath; I have used the 15-volume, Boston edition of 1861 ff. (not to be confused with the 7-volume, London edition); this collection hereafter is referred to as "Bacon, *Works.*" In recent appraisals, Loren Eiseley, *Francis Bacon and the Modern Dilemma* (Lincoln, Nebr., 1962) is very favorable, while René Dubos, *The Dreams of Reason: Science and Utopias* (New York, 1961) is critical of the Baconian "cult of science."
[53] Bacon, *Works* 8: p. 113.
[54] *Ibid.* 5: p. 398.

[55] Quoted in Farrington, *op. cit.* (see fn. 52), p. 68.
[56] Bacon, *Works* 8: p. 142.
[57] *Ibid.* 13: pp. 144–156. On Prometheus, *cf.* earlier, chap. II.
[58] On the role of serpents in legends of this type, see earlier, chap. II.
[59] Bacon, *Works* 13: p. 150.
[60] On the contradiction in Bacon between primitivism and progressism, *cf.* Farrington, *op. cit.* (see fn. 52), pp. 76, 169–170.
[61] Bacon, *Works* 9: p. 39.

The philosopher here felt it necessary to defend himself against possible imputations of impiety by asserting that, while the term of life may rest in the hands of Providence, this does not rule out the advantages to be derived from preventive measures.[62]

. . . although to a Christian making for the Land of Promise the world is but a wilderness, yet even while we travel in the wilderness to have our shoes and garments (that is our bodies, which are as the clothing of the soul) not worn out by the way, must be accounted as a gift of divine grace.[63]

The zealous prolongevitist still seems to have felt defensive in the face of orthodox religious teachings implying the unimportance of the things of this world; in his *History of Life and Death,* he added another rebuttal.

. . . though the life of man is only a mass and accumulation of sins and sorrows, and they who aspire to eternity set little value on life; yet even we Christians should not despise the continuance of works of charity. Besides, the beloved disciple survived the rest, and many of the Fathers, especially holy monks and hermits, were long-lived.[64]

The reformer went on, in the *Advancement of Learning,* to criticize physicians for neglecting the prolongation of life, the "principal part of their art."

. . . the lengthening of the thread of life itself, and the postponement for a time of that death which gradually steals on by natural dissolution and the decay of age, is a subject which no physician has handled in proportion to its dignity.[65]

Bacon, somewhat loftily, gave four admonitions to the profession as guidance in this new field.[66] First, that, to date, all works on the subject have been unsound; Aristotle's contribution was only of slight value, while more modern writers (apparently, the alchemists and iatrochemists) were vain and superstitious. Second, that naive efforts to preserve natural warmth and moisture do more harm than good. Third, and perhaps the most apt, that prolongevity is a long and complex undertaking:

. . . men should cease from trifling, nor be so credulous as to imagine that so great a work as this of delaying and turning back the course of nature can be effected by a morning draught or by the use of some precious drug; by potable gold, or essence of pearls, or suchlike toys.

And fourth, that it is necessary to distinguish between the regimen for health and that for longevity, for that which exhilarates the body and spirit is not necessarily conducive to long life.

In Solomon's House, Bacon's imaginary Academy of Science, we find the savants busily engaged in the struggle for health and longevity. Not only did they have special foods and medicines for the rapid cure of dis-

ease,[67] but also, ". . . amongst them we have a water which we call Water of Paradise, being, by that we do to it, made very sovereign for health, and prolongation of life." [68] In addition, mention is made of deep caves, which because of their atmospheric properties possessed virtue in healing the ill and prolonging life [69]; and there were special bathing facilities which restored "the very juice and substance" of the human body.[70]

Among the most remarkable features of Solomon's House were the experiments performed on animals:

We have also . . . all sorts of beasts and birds, which we use . . . for dissections and trials; that thereby we may take light what may be wrought upon the body of man. Wherein we find many strange effects; as continuing life in them, though divers parts, which you account vital, be perished and taken forth; resuscitating of some that seem dead in appearance; and the like.[71]

This passage is notable not only for its prediction of experimental medicine, but also because it reveals a new attitude towards death, a loss of awe and fear regarding it and a willingness to apply scientific methods to the very boundary zone between life and death. The medicine of the Enlightenment was characterized by a compulsion to resuscitate the "dead" and to attempt to replace vital organs [72]; and ultimately this concern was to help to bring about, in the present century, such highly useful developments as efficient artificial respiration, cardiac massage, the heart-lung machine, the artificial kidney, and intra-cardiac surgery.

Bacon's own endeavor to formulate a scientific basis for prolongevity was presented in his *History of Life and Death*.[73] This was an essential component of his "Great Instauration," the first part of which was the *Advancement of Learning* and the second, the *Novum organum;* the third part was the *Natural and Experimental History* consisting of "histories" of all sorts of natural phenomena: the winds, density and rarity, sulphur and mercury, etc. Among these latter treatises was the "history" of life and death, a diffusely organized compendium of aphorisms, data, and "explications" which show evidence of wide reading and shrewd observation of the everyday scene. But there is little in

---

[62] *Ibid.,* pp. 29–30.
[63] *Ibid.,* p. 39.
[64] *Ibid.* 10: p. 11.
[65] *Ibid.* 9: p. 29.
[66] *Ibid.,* pp. 40–41.

[67] *Ibid.* 5: p. 366.
[68] *Ibid.,* p. 400. *Cf.* the fountain-of-youth legends; see earlier, chap. III.
[69] *Ibid.,* pp. 398–399.
[70] *Ibid.,* p. 401.
[71] *Ibid.,* pp. 401–402. *Cf.* Saul Jarcho, transl., "Experiments of Doctor Joseph Zambeccari Concerning the Excision of Various Organs from Different Living Animals (1680)," *Bull. Hist. of Medicine* 9 (1941): pp. 311–331.
[72] The Humane Societies of the eighteenth century were dedicated to a virtual crusade on behalf of resuscitation; see Elizabeth H. Thomson, "The Role of Physicians in the Humane Societies of the Eighteenth Century," *Bull. Hist. of Medicine* 37 (1963): pp. 43–51.
[73] I have used Francis Bacon, *History, Naturall and Experimentall, of Life and Death,* William Rawley, transl. (London, 1638); hereafter referred to as "Bacon, *History.*" *Cf.* Bacon, *Works* 10: pp. 7–176.

it to suggest sustained and systematic observation and experiment, and the tone is more akin to that of Avicenna's *Canon of Medicine* or even Pliny's *Natural History* than to an advanced work like Harvey's *On the Motion of the Heart*. It is one more example of the fact that Bacon was more impressive as a prophet of science than in doing the scientific work itself.

Both the theory of aging and the regimen of pro-longevity set forth by Bacon were largely derivative; as with Aristotle and Galen, his explanation of senescence was based on vitalism and humoralism.[74] Although he disdained the terms "innate heat" and "innate moisture,"[75] he replaced them with a similar concept, that of "spirits" which consisted of a miraculous combination of flame and air.[76] These spirits, he stated, are essential to the functioning of the body, but, because they are akin to combustion, they tend to dry the fluids and burn up the oily substances of the body; moreover, the spirits tend to escape into the surrounding air.[77] The result is that the nature of old age is the same as in the traditional hypotheses: the spirits become rarified, the oily fluids become watery, the blood becomes cold, and there is an excess of the phlegmatic (cold and wet) and the melancholic (cold and dry) humors.[78]

To postpone the decline of the body forces, the philosopher had a vast number of suggestions, bearing out his admonition that prolongevity is a long and complex operation. There were three principal aims. First, the spirits must be conserved and their actions modified: they may be "condensed" by certain drugs (e.g., opium and nitre), their escape may be blocked by coating with oil the pores of the skin, and their harmful effects on the blood may be decreased by baths (which cool the blood).[79] Secondly, one may attempt to aid those processes which restore and regenerate the body: for example, certain herbs strengthen the vital organs, while a proper regimen (diet, exercise, etc.) helps to improve the digestion and assimilation of food.[80] Finally, there are efforts directed at rejuvenation: thus, overly dry parts may be softened and moistened by massage and special baths, while periodically one may take herbs and purgatives for the "purging away of old juice and supplying of new juice."[81]

The significance of the *History of Life and Death* is that it brought great prestige to prolongevitism. To be sure, the work offered nothing very new either in

theory or practice, and its approach was not abreast of the new physiology of Harvey or Descartes; it was, however, a workmanlike performance quite up to the level of most clinical literature of the time. Moreover, it gave to prolongevitism the endorsement of an illustrious name; already in 1652, a disciple of Descartes was defending the master's interest in longevity by citing the example of Bacon.[82] The fame of the English philosopher grew to be almost boundless, for his vision of Solomon's House stimulated the formation of the Royal Society, which, after the epoch-making achievements of Newton, became the model for all scientific societies. Newton himself was in many respects a Baconian and helped to stamp the impress of that philosopher on eighteenth-century science. Bacon's concern with lengthening life was well known, and, since his day, virtually every work on prolongevity has mentioned his commendation of this "most noble" subject.

BLOOD TRANSFUSION [83]

As a postscript to the discussion of Descartes and Bacon, a few words may be added concerning the part played by prolongevitism in the early development of one of the most valuable techniques of modern medicine —the transfusion of blood. Bacon, as we have seen, urged in the *New Atlantis* that trials be made of the feasibility of removing and replacing vital organs, and in the *History of Life and Death* he speculated about the beneficial effects on the aged of substituting new body "juices" for old. At nearly the same time, the physiological basis for transfusion was provided by Harvey's theory of the vascular circulation. It followed that an attempt should be made to rejuvenate the aging organism by transfusing it with youthful blood. Unfortunately, such procedures were premature for clinical application, because the necessary techniques of antisepsis and blood-typing were not yet available.

The first successful blood transfusions in animals (dogs) were performed by the English physician and physiologist Richard Lower in 1650, and the new skill quickly was applied to trials of rejuvenation. Thus, we read in the *Philosophical Transactions* of the Royal So-

---

[74] On the gerontological theories of Aristotle, Galen, and Avicenna, see earlier, chap. II.

[75] Bacon, *History*, p. 172.

[76] *Ibid.*, pp. 344–346, 359–360, 390–391, 431 ff. The Baconian and similar concepts of "spirits" are analyzed by Allen G. Debus, "The Paracelsian Aerial Niter." *Isis* 55 (1964): pp. 43–61.

[77] *Ibid.*, pp. 28, 43–46, 382, 433.

[78] *Ibid.*, pp. 371–372.

[79] *Ibid.*, pp. 183 ff.

[80] *Ibid.*, pp. 277 ff.

[81] *Ibid.*, pp. 324 ff.

[82] Adam, *Vie* (see fn. 17), pp. 581–582.

[83] There is a valuable collection of material on transfusion experiments in the seventeenth century in John Lowthorp, ed., *The Philosophical Transactions and Collections to the End of the Year 1700, Abridg'd and Dispos'd under General Heads* (2nd ed., London, 1716) 3: pp. 225–235. On the French experience, there is a provocative reinterpretation by Harcourt Brown, "Jean Denis and Transfusion of Blood: Paris, 1667–1668," *Isis* 39 (1948): pp. 15–29. On the general history of blood transfusion, the present author has used N. S. R. Maluf, "History of Blood Transfusion," *Jour. Hist. of Medicine* 9 (1954): pp. 59–107 and Leo M. Zimmerman and Katherine M. Howell, "History of Blood Transfusion," *Annals of Medical History* 4 (1932): pp. 415–433; two other studies are Heinrich Buess, "Die Bluttransfusion," *Ciba Zeitschrift* 7 (1956): pp. 2610–2644 and Geoffrey Keynes, "The History of Blood Transfusion," *Science News* (Penguin Books) 3 (1947).

ciety of the experiment by Coxen in which "an old mongrel curr, all over-run with the mainge" was transfused with "14–16 oz." of blood from a young spaniel and was "perfectly cured." [84] A similar investigation was reported as follows:

Mr. Gayant transfused the blood of a young dog into the veins of an old, which two hours after, did leap and frisk; whereas he was almost blind with age, and could hardly stir before.[85]

From Italy in 1668 came the report that the blood of a lamb had had a marvelous restorative effect on a decrepit, thirteen-year-old spaniel.[86]

Meanwhile, the idea had been taken up by Jean Denis, a Paris physician, who attracted attention by a public demonstration of the revitalization of a mangy old canine by blood from a healthy young animal; a like test was carried out on an ancient horse.[87] A supporter of Denis wrote to the *Journal des savants* advocating the new method as a cure for all sorts of diseases and for rejuvenating the aged, and, during 1667, Denis performed the first human blood transfusion.[88] We know of five cases in which the procedure was tried; curiously enough, none of these were senescent. Undoubtedly, the infusions would have been applied, sooner or later, to aged persons, but Denis' work was brought to an early end by the sudden death of one of his patients; this led to a lawsuit and finally to a moratorium by the powerful Faculty of Medicine on further experiments. Despite a few sporadic, ineffectual efforts by others, the further evolution of transfusion was delayed until the early nineteenth century.

THE EIGHTEENTH CENTURY

FRANKLIN [89]

Benjamin Franklin's most explicit comment on prolongevity serves as the epigraph for this chapter; de-

spite its brevity, it is a remarkable statement, and it illustrates some of the tendencies in eighteenth-century life and thought which prepared the way for the radical prolongevitism of Godwin and Condorcet. The most striking part of the passage is the assertion that, because of the progress of science, the length of life may be extended beyond the antediluvian standard; and this vision of a drastic increase in longevity came from a man noted for his practical common sense. Nothing could demonstrate better Franklin's freedom from preconceptions which had loomed large in the thinking of previous Western prolongevitists. Primitivism no longer carried any weight, as it had with Roger Bacon and even with Francis Bacon; Franklin looked entirely to the future. And the dogma of the fall of man, which still had inhibited Descartes and Francis Bacon, no longer influenced Franklin, for his religious views were founded on reason rather than revelation. While earlier writers carefully had kept their aspirations within the bounds of the Patriarchal life spans, Franklin could speak of surpassing them.

In regard to the "rapid progress" which science was making in extending "the power of man over matter," no one could speak with greater authority than Franklin; he was associated with some of the most spectacular scientific and technological achievements of all time. To his contemporaries, the most symbolic of these attainments was Franklin's own invention—the lightning rod. Thunder and lightning always had been associated with the realm of the supernatural and the divine, and, for bringing this dreaded force under control, the American was hailed by Condorcet as "the modern Prometheus." [90] Electricity was not actually put to work until the next century, but, when that era arrived, it owed much to Franklin's fundamental research in the subject.[91] Franklin also was in touch with another epoch-making technological innovation—the steam engine.[92] Then there was "the new art of flying" which greatly excited the American diplomat in 1783.[93] Like prolongevity, flying had long been a theme of folklore and the object of apologist scorn, as in the legend of Daedalus and Icarus; now, the successful ascent in balloons by Montgolfier and others moved Franklin to salute "a discovery of great importance, and what may possibly give a new turn to human affairs." The scientist and statesman also was in close touch with medical advances; he was, for example, a strong advocate of inoculation for

---

[84] Lowthorp, *op. cit.* (see fn. 83), p. 229.

[85] *Idem.*

[86] *Ibid.,* p. 230.

[87] *Idem* and Brown, *op. cit.* (see fn. 83), p. 19.

[88] Brown, *op. cit.* (see fn. 83), pp. 19 ff.

[89] The standard biography is Carl Van Doren, *Benjamin Franklin* (New York, 1938). Also useful is Bernard Fay, *Franklin: the Apostle of Modern Times* (Boston, 1929). A valuable edition of the autobiography is Max Farrand, ed., *Benjamin Franklin's Memoirs: Parallel Text Edition* (Berkeley, 1949). The authoritative study of Franklin's role in eighteenth-century science is I. Bernard Cohen, *Franklin and Newton,* Mem. Amer. Philos. Soc. 43 (Philadelphia, 1956) ; by the same author, there is a survey of Franklin's personality and activities, *Benjamin Franklin: his Contribution to the American Tradition* (Indianapolis, 1953). Earlier collections of Franklin's writings by Jared Sparks (1840), John Bigelow (1887), and Albert Henry Smyth (1905) are being superseded by Leonard W. Labaree and Whitfield J. Bell, Jr., eds., *The Papers of Benjamin Franklin* (New Haven, 1959 ff.). The engaging essay by Carl Becker in the *Dictionary of American Biography* has been reprinted, with an introduction by Julian P. Boyd, as *Benjamin Franklin: a Biographical Sketch* (Ithaca, 1946).

[90] Albert H. Smyth, ed., *The Writings of Benjamin Franklin* (New York, 1905) 1: p. 196.

[91] *Cf.* I. Bernard Cohen, ed., *Benjamin Franklin's Experiments: a New Edition of Franklin's Experiments and Observations on Electricity* (Cambridge, Mass., 1941).

[92] Paul Mantoux, *The Industrial Revolution in the Eighteenth Century,* Marjorie Vernon, transl. (rev. ed., London, 1928), p. 331.

[93] On Franklin's interest in balloons, see Edward E. Hale and Edward E. Hale, Jr., *Franklin in France* (2 v., Boston, 1888) 2: pp. 268–289.

smallpox, one of the first effective weapons of preventive medicine.[94]

The prospect of sweeping advances in science was, for Franklin, not without a melancholy side, for it "occasions my regretting sometimes that I was born so soon." Thus, the idea of progress not only supported the belief that prolongevity was possible but also enhanced its desirability; for it canceled out the ancient Epicurean doctrine of the "fullness of pleasure," according to which life held the possibility of only a limited number of happy experiences.[95] Descartes, as we have seen, had such exalted hopes for science and philosophy that he yearned to live long enough to see them become reality; consequently, he became anxious about the brevity of life expectancy and applied himself to medicine in order to prolong life. Franklin's expectations for the future were even greater, and he too felt very keenly the desire to live on to see the wonders to come.[96] This feeling was expressed in a half-serious, half-jocular passage in a letter to Dr. Jacques Barbeu-Dubourg, discussing, among other things, the revival, by the sun, of flies which had been "drowned" in wine.

I wish it were possible, from this instance, to invent a method of embalming drowned persons, in such a manner that they may be recalled to life at any period, however distant; for having a very ardent desire to see and observe the state of America a hundred years hence, I should prefer to any ordinary death, the being immersed in a cask of Madeira wine, with a few friends, till that time, to be then recalled to life by the solar warmth of my dear country. But since in all probability we live in an age too early and too near the infancy of science, to hope to see an art brought in our time to its perfection, I must for the present content myself with the treat, which you are so kind as to promise me, of the resurrection of a fowl or a turkey cock.[97]

Franklin's speculation about suspended animation had a genuine scientific basis, for the eighteenth century had seen the discovery of "anabiosis," a condition of the organism in which it is deprived of all signs of life and yet still can be resuscitated.[98] The phenomenon first had been noted in microbes (dried rotifers) by Leeuwenhoek in 1702, and, as further studies were made, a good bit of discussion was aroused concerning the nature of life and death.[99] Observations of this sort fit in very

well with the tendency of the Enlightenment to do away with the mystery and awe associated with death; the *philosophes* were consistently interested in resuscitation, as, for example, in the same letter from Franklin to his close friend Dr. Barbeu-Dubourg:

Your observations on the causes of death and the experiments which you propose for recalling to life those who appear to be killed by lightning, demonstrate equally your sagacity and your humanity. It appears that the doctrines of life and death in general are yet but little understood.[100]

The American went on to speculate rather uncritically about alleged cases of anabiosis: a toad which becomes petrified in sand and rock may live for "we know not how many ages," while, as already mentioned, flies drowned in wine are "capable of being revived by the rays of the sun."

The great, eighteenth-century anatomist and surgeon John Hunter had similar ideas and thought of applications to prolongevity; in 1766 he froze several carp and then thawed them very slowly, but, to his disappointment, they failed to revive.

Till this time I had imagined that it might be possible to prolong life to any period by freezing a person in the frigid zone, as I thought all action and waste would cease until the body was thawed. I thought that if a man would give up the last ten years of his life to this kind of alternate oblivion and action, it might be prolonged to a thousand years: and by getting himself thawed every hundred years, he might learn what had happened during his frozen condition.[101]

Such speculation was very premature, but, in our own day, the discovery in 1948 (actually first reported by Jean Rostand in 1946) of the protective effects of glycerol has allowed the production, by freezing, of anabiosis in mammals (rats and hamsters), and the extension of the technique to humans seems probable.[102]

---

[94] On Franklin and medicine, see William Pepper, *The Medical Side of Benjamin Franklin* (Philadelphia, 1911); Theodore Diller, *Franklin's Contribution to Medicine* (Brooklyn, 1912); and Benjamin Franklin, *Some Account of the Pennsylvania Hospital*, I. Bernard Cohen, ed. (Baltimore, 1954).

[95] On the Epicureans, see earlier, chap. II.

[96] On the desire to see the future; *cf.* Francis Bacon's remark, "I have lost much time with this age; I would be glad to recover it with posterity"; quoted in Eiseley, *op. cit.* (see fn. 52), pp. 25–26.

[97] Pepper, *op. cit.* (see fn. 94), pp. 61–62.

[98] On the history of anabiosis, see D. Keilin, "The Problem of Anabiosis or Latent Life: History and Current Concept," *Proc. Royal Society*, B **150** (1959): pp. 149–191.

[99] *Ibid.*, pp. 150–157. *Cf.* "the Endymion theme," see earlier, chap. III.

[100] Pepper, *op. cit.* (see fn. 94), p. 61. On Enlightenment interest in resuscitation, see Thomson, *op. cit.* (see fn. 72). On a non-meliorist plane, an example of materialist tendencies of the time was the preservation, by the family, of the body of Madame Necker (d. 1794) in a stone basin filled with alcohol; see J. Christopher Herold, *Mistress to an Age: a Life of Madame de Staël* (Indianapolis and New York, 1958), pp. 50–51, 471–472.

[101] John Hunter, *Lectures on the Principles of Surgery* (Philadelphia, 1841), p. 76.

[102] A. S. Parkes, "Preservation of Tissue *in vitro* for the Study of Ageing," in G. E. W. Wolstenholme and Cecilia M. O'Connor, eds., *General Aspects of Ageing*, Ciba Foundation Colloquia on Ageing **1** (Boston, 1955): pp. 162–169. It would seem that the ability to produce anabiosis in humans might have extensive use, for, in this way, a person afflicted with a hopeless disease (e.g., cancer) could be preserved in a frozen condition until such time as a cure might be discovered. R. C. W. Ettinger proposes early application of this idea in *The Prospect of Immortality* (New York, 1964), "The Frozen Christian," *Christian Century* **82** (1965): pp. 1313–1315 and "Science and Immortality," *Yale Scientific Magazine* **40**, 7 (1966): pp. 5–8, 20. *Cf.* the newsletter described in chap. III, fn. 81.

GODWIN [103]

The ideas of Godwin and Condorcet mark the culmination of eighteenth-century prolongevitism. Both were tremendously excited by the French Revolution, and their chief works appeared at almost the same time in the early 1790's. There are several other areas of strong agreement between the two: both, for example, were essentially religious in spirit although professedly atheist, and both were deeply committed to the idea of progress and the perfectability of man; in brief, they are excellent examples of the truth of Becker's thesis that much of the Enlightenment represented a secularized form of Christian eschatology. They also illustrate the shortcomings of Becker's analysis of the attitude of the *philosophes* towards death: where Becker felt that the Enlightenment's solution of the problem of death consisted of the posthumous cult of the hero, there also was a powerful tendency, as has been seen in Descartes, Bacon, and Franklin, to seek a material victory over death by the prolongation of life. With Godwin and Condorcet this theme becomes unmistakable, for they sought a virtual immortality on earth.

At the same time, there are significant differences between the two thinkers; they characterize, in some respects, two contrasting trends within the Enlightenment. Godwin considered the individual to be the chief agent of progress, while Condorcet saw society as the main carrier of progress. In the slogan, "Liberty, equality, fraternity," Godwin would prefer liberty, and Condorcet would emphasize fraternity; one was a founder of philosophical anarchism, the other of sociology. To Godwin, the essential for human advance was "individual independence"; to Condorcet, organized scientific research. As to the type of salvation they aimed for, they also represent divergent tendencies. In the heaven of traditional religion there were two sorts of blessings: first, and more important, there was freedom from sin, i.e., the moral evils of this world, and secondly, there was liberation from material deprivations, i.e., poverty, disease, and death. Godwin was more in keeping with traditional religious teachings in making salvation from sin the primary task, while Condorcet was more revolutionary in stressing the primacy of salvation from material ills. The English reformer believed that ethics was the most powerful means for achieving the perfectability of man; the Frenchman looked instead to the natural sciences.

From Godwin's *Enquiry Concerning Political Justice,* published in 1793, we may single out several of the principles which led him to prolongevitism.[104] First, there is the power of reason [105]: according to Godwin, "Man is a rational being," [106] and the philosopher pushed to extremes this idea of the supremacy of reason over the emotions. It followed that, "Truth is omnipotent," for, if man is essentially rational, he will be sure to recognize truth from falsehood. And this victory of truth is vital, for the mind "possesses an undisputed empire over the conduct." [107] From these assumptions, there evolved the belief in the perfectability of man.[108] Because of the power of reason and the omnipotence of truth, there will be a perpetual improvement in knowledge, and that knowledge will be accepted by mankind and applied to the improvement of the race.

From his doctrines of individualism, the power of reason, and the perfectability of man, Godwin deduced that it should be possible to lengthen life by increasing the sway of "mind over matter." [109] The philosopher was careful to dissociate his system of prolongevity from those of Francis Bacon, Franklin, and Condorcet:

> These authors . . . have inclined to rest their hopes, rather upon the growing power of art, than, as is here done, upon the immediate and unavoidable operation of an improved intellect.[110]

What Godwin conceived was the "potential omnipotence" of the mind of the individual over the matter of his own body. Because of the perfectability of man, such control would be advanced inexorably until death itself might be overcome [111]: "In a word, why may not man be one day immortal?" [112]

On behalf of this mind-over-matter prolongevity, Godwin cited the sort of phenomena which today are included in psychosomatic medicine.[113] The arrival of good news may cure some bodily indispositions, and, on the contrary, unhappy mental impressions may produce a "broken heart" or even bring about organic disease. People who are busy and active resist harmful influences sufficient to reduce the indolent to illness.

> I walk twenty miles, full of ardour, and with a motive that engrosses my soul, and I arrive as fresh and alert as when I began my journey. Emotion, excited by some unexpected word, by a letter that is delivered to us, occasions the most extraordinary revolutions in our frame. . . . There is noth-

103 A charming introduction to Godwin is H. N. Brailsford, *Shelley, Godwin and Their Circle* (London, 1913). A competent survey of Godwin's life and work is David Fleisher, *William Godwin: a Study in Liberalism* (London, 1951). The older, standard biography is C. Kegan Paul, *William Godwin: his Friends and Contemporaries* (2 v., London, 1876).

104 The most useful edition is William Godwin, *Enquiry Concerning Political Justice, and its Influence on Morals and Happiness,* third edition with variant readings of the first and second, F. E. L. Priestley, ed. (3 v., Toronto, 1946); hereafter referred to as "Godwin, *Enquiry.*"
105 *Ibid.* 1: pp. 52–95.
106 *Ibid.,* p. 88.
107 *Ibid.,* p. 92.
108 *Ibid.,* pp. 92–95.
109 *Ibid.* 2: pp. 519–529.
110 *Ibid.,* p. 520.
111 *Cf.* Thomas Aquinas on immortality as a result of the rule of mind over body; see earlier, chap. II.
112 Godwin, *Enquiry* 3: p. 224.
113 *Ibid.* 2: pp. 521–523.

ing of which the physician is more frequently aware, than of the power of the mind in assisting or retarding convalescence.[114]

Where Godwin would differ from present-day psychosomatic theory is that he considered these phenomena to be quite subject to conscious control, whereas today the role of the subconscious is preeminent.

From these examples of emotional influences on bodily health, Godwin proceeded to speculate about mental hygiene as a cause of long life.

A habit peculiarly favourable to corporeal vigour, is chearfulness. Every time that our mind becomes morbid, vacant or melancholy, our external frame falls into disorder. Littleness of thought is the brother of death. But chearfulness gives new elasticity to our limbs, and circulation to our juices.[115]

These opinions led the reformer to frame a hypothesis as to the moral and emotional causes of senescence.

Why is it that a mature man loses that elasticity of limb, which characterizes the heedless gaiety of youth? The origin of this appears to be, that he desists from youthful habits. . . . He is visited and vexed with the cares that rise out of our mistaken institutions, and his heart is no longer satisfied and gay. His limbs become stiff, unwieldy and awkward. This is the forerunner of old age and death.[116]

It followed that right thinking and right living should increase longevity, and the recipe for immortality is "chearfulness, clearness of conception and benevolence." [117] Moreover, the belief in prolongevity is a factor making for these desirable qualities; we become sick, and we die, partly because we expect such a fate and consent to it; but if we had faith in prolongevity, our more sanguine temper would prolong our lives.[118]

Beyond this, Godwin pictured a gradual extension of voluntary control over bodily functions, for the perfectability of man means "to attain as nearly as possible, to the perfectly voluntary state." [119] The workings of the circulatory system, for instance, are at present not generally subject to voluntary control; nonetheless, it is a common observation that "certain thoughts and states of the thinking faculty" affect the operations of this system, causing, for example, palpitations of the heart. Furthermore, some persons already possess conscious control over certain bodily actions which in the generality of mankind are not subject to mental intervention. Therefore, as man perfects himself, he may expect to bring his body under the rule of mind:

If volition can now do something, why should it not go on to do still more and more? There is no principle of reason less liable to question than this, that, if we have in any

respect a little power now, and if mind be essentially progressive, that power may, and, barring any extraordinary concussions of nature, infallibly will, extend beyond any bounds we are able to prescribe to it.[120]

First sleep will be overcome, then death itself: ". . . before death can be banished, we must banish sleep, death's image. Sleep is one of the most conspicuous infirmities of the human frame." [121]

These ideas about the prolongation of life found a quick rejoinder in Thomas Malthus' *Essay on the Principle of Population*, published in 1798, a work inspired by opposition to the *philosophes* and subtitled *On the Speculations of Mr. Godwin, M. Condorcet, and Other Writers*.[122] Malthus did not deny the existence of the psychosomatic phenomena listed by Godwin, but he considered them the result of "mental stimulants," and he believed such stimulants could have only a limited effectiveness.[123] He agreed that a man in high spirits might walk twenty miles without feeling fatigue, but if he were set to walk another twenty miles and then another, ultimately, no matter how great his motivation, muscle would be seen to prevail over mind. Similarly, in a mild illness "mental stimulants" might have some influence, but of what avail were such factors in severe diseases like smallpox or the plague? As to the voluntary control of bodily functions, Malthus admitted there might be a few persons able to perform feats of this sort, but he considered such performances to be mere "tricks" not applicable to any good purpose. The conclusion is that neither "mental stimulants" nor "tricks" can be viewed as potential means for a significant extension of longevity:

There is certainly a sufficiently marked difference in the various characters of which we have some knowledge, relative to the energies of their minds, their benevolent pursuits, etc. to enable us to judge, whether the operations of intellect have any decided effect in prolonging the duration of human life. It is certain, that no decided effect of this kind has yet been observed.[124]

In Malthusian apologism, the mainstay, of course, was the hypothesis of overpopulation, a doctrine which would make prolongevity definitely undesirable. According to Malthus, the population tends to increase in geometric ratio, while the supply of foodstuffs increases only arithmetically; therefore, society always is in a state of overpopulation, and poverty and disease are virtually inevitable.[125] In this view, the prolongation of life, far from being a blessing, actually would aggravate the situa-

---

[114] *Ibid.*, p. 521.
[115] Godwin, *Enquiry* 2: p. 522.
[116] *Idem.*
[117] *Ibid.* 3: p. 225.
[118] *Ibid.* 2: pp. 526–527 and 3: p. 227.
[119] *Ibid.* 2: pp. 523, 525.

[120] *Ibid.* 3: p. 225.
[121] *Ibid.*, p. 226. *Cf.* sleep in the story of Gilgamesh; see earlier, chap. II.
[122] Thomas Robert Malthus, *An Essay on the Principle of Population, as it Affects the Future Improvement of Society, with Remarks on the Speculations of Mr. Godwin, M. Condorcet, and Other Writers* (London, 1798) ; this work hereafter is referred to as "Malthus, *Essay.*"
[123] *Ibid.*, pp. 220–239.
[124] *Ibid.*, p. 237.
[125] *Ibid.*, pp. 13–17 and *passim.*

tion by producing a still greater surplus population.[126]

Godwin had been aware of an earlier version of Malthusianism, an essay published by Robert Wallace in 1761,[127] and he had formulated three possible means of circumventing the problem. The most fanciful, perhaps, was the idea that, since the perfectability of man means the increasing sway of reason, it follows that, in the course of human progress, sex will become a matter of little interest.

> One tendency of a cultivated and virtuous mind is to diminish our eagerness for the gratification of the senses. . . . We soon learn to despise the mere animal function. . . . The men therefore whom we are supposing to exist, when the earth shall refuse itself to a more extended population, will probably cease to propagate. The whole will be a people of men, and not of children. Generation will not succeed generation, nor truth have, in a certain degree, to recommence her career every thirty years.[128]

This belief that, with progress, man should become more reasonable and, therefore, less concerned with a primitive function like sex, exerted a strong influence in forming nineteenth-century Victorianism and still was being propounded in the twentieth by the paragon of rationalism, George Bernard Shaw.[129] Malthus, though a clergyman, would have none of it and wrote eloquently in defense of the sexual instinct.[130] Godwin, meanwhile, had in reserve two other plans: "improvements" in agriculture and industry would delay the onset of overpopulation for many centuries and, if that failed, society could resort to birth control.[131] Malthus, however, felt there was little amplitude for technological progress,[132] and, unlike the neo-Malthusians, he was opposed (on moral grounds) to birth control.[133]

In assessing the significance of Godwin's prolongevitism, it may be said that the line of thought which he pursued has not been very influential. To be sure, Godwin's ideas still are familiar, both in the supernatural form of Christian Science and the natural variant of Shaw. But his advocacy of an "intellectual" and individualistic sort of medicine has not found many followers, for it has been undermined by the same factors which swept away the foundations of the personal, prolongevity hygiene of the Cornaro tradition. The progress of medicine since Godwin's day has been in the development of impersonal, standardized therapy with drugs, sera, radiation, etc. combined with complex social methods of public health. Medical science has followed

the path of Francis Bacon, Franklin, and Condorcet in putting its faith in "the growing power of art," the very path from which Godwin was so careful to dissociate himself.

CONDORCET [134]

Condorcet's history of human progress, published in 1795, may serve as an illustration of Becker's thesis that the *philosophes* owed much to medieval Christianity.[135] The similarity is striking between the organization of this work and Otto of Freising's *Two Cities,* compiled by the German bishop in 1146.[136] Otto dealt with all history in eight books: the first begins with Adam and Eve, the second includes the Greeks and the Roman republic, in the third Christianity appears, and the fourth, fifth, and sixth carry the story to about 1085. Otto's book seven dealt with "our own times," while book eight, the most interesting of all, depicted the glories of the future with the resurrection and judgment and the salvation of mankind from sin and death.

Condorcet divided history into ten stages: the first was the era of primitive tribes, while the ninth concerns the seventeenth and eighteenth centuries up to the French Revolution. The tenth stage of Condorcet, like the eighth of Otto, is devoted to the wonders of the future; but where Otto spoke of earthly history as a tragedy and looked to the other world for salvation, Condorcet saw history as a victorious progress and visualized a virtual heaven on earth. Otto thought of the world as in extreme old age and about to end; Condorcet viewed it as just reaching maturity and with its greatest prosperity yet to come.

In the march of progress envisioned by Condorcet, the prolongation of life had a major place, as he set forth in the famous passage:

> Would it be absurd then to suppose that this perfection of the human species might be capable of indefinite progress; that the day will come when death will be due only to extraordinary accidents or to the decay of the vital forces, and that ultimately, the average span between birth and decay will have no assignable value? Certainly man will not become immortal, but will not the interval between the first breath that he draws and the time when in the natural course of events, without disease or accident, he expires, increase indefinitely? [137]

[126] *Ibid.,* p. 171.

[127] Robert Wallace, *Various Prospects of Mankind, Nature and Providence* (London, 1761).

[128] Godwin, *Enquiry* 2: pp. 527–528.

[129] George Bernard Shaw, *Back to Methuselah* (New York, 1921).

[130] Malthus, *Essay,* pp. 210–215.

[131] Godwin, *Enquiry* 2: pp. 515–519.

[132] E.g., Malthus attacked Adam Smith for advocating industrialization as a means to raise living standards; Malthus, *Essay,* pp. 303–326.

[133] *Ibid.,* p. 154.

[134] A good, brief biography and useful bibliography are in J. Salwyn Schapiro, *Condorcet and the Rise of Liberalism* (New York, 1934), pp. 66–109, 284–286; see also, Frank E. Manuel, *The Prophets of Paris* (Cambridge, Mass., 1962), pp. 53–102. The best edition of the works is Antoine-Nicolas de Condorcet, *Œuvres,* A. Condorcet O'Connor and M. F. Arago, eds. (12 v., Paris, 1847–1849).

[135] A scholarly translation is Antoine-Nicolas de Condorcet, *Sketch for a Historical Picture of the Progress of the Human Mind,* June Barraclough, transl., Library of Ideas (New York, 1955); hereafter referred to as "Condorcet, *Progress.*"

[136] Otto, Bishop of Freising, *The Two Cities,* C. C. Mierow, transl. (New York, 1928).

[137] Condorcet, *Progress,* p. 200.

The philosopher-mathematician went on to indicate that, if he was not thinking of immortality itself, he was coming very close to it.

In truth, this average span of life which we suppose will increase indefinitely as time passes, may grow in conformity either with a law such that it continually approaches a limitless length but without ever reaching it, or with a law such that through the centuries it reaches a length greater than any determinate quantity that we may assign to it as its limit.

The three main foundations for Condorcet's prolongevitism were the improvement of the environment, the inheritance of acquired characteristics, and the advancement of medical science. The *philosophe* was highly interested in public health, the branch of medicine most closely related to his own efforts for social and political reform. Like the nineteenth-century sanitarians, he felt that disease could be blamed largely on impure air, overwork, an unwise diet, and violent passions.[188] He was particularly fond of inveighing against the indolent luxury and intemperance of the rich and the excessive cares and anxieties of the poor. As these evils will be overcome by "the progress of reason and of the social order," life expectancy will increase:

No one can doubt that, as preventitive medicine improves and food and housing become healthier, as a way of life is established that develops our physical powers by exercise without ruining them by excess, as the two most virulent causes of deterioration, misery and excessive wealth, are eliminated, the average length of human life will be increased and a better health and a stronger physical constitution will be ensured.[189]

In Condorcet's opinion, these improvements in the human physique would be enhanced further with each generation by the inheritance of acquired characteristics.[140] Like Roger Bacon, he applied to prolongevity the doctrine which has come to be known as Lamarckism, in honor of the French naturalist who used it to build a theory of evolution.[141] Nearly all early workers in biology had accepted the principle that those traits which an organism develops under the influence of the environment are passed on to its descendants. As Condorcet put it:

But are not our physical faculties and the strength, dexterity and acuteness of our senses, to be numbered among the qualities whose perfection in the individual may be transmitted? Observation of the various breeds of domestic animals inclines us to believe that they are, and we can confirm this by direct observation of the human race.[142]

The reformer felt that even intellectual and moral faculties might be passed on to succeeding generations, thereby further perfecting the race.[143] Condorcet's speculations along this line excited the emulation of Cabanis, the great physician-philosopher of the early 1800's, who in his writings referred again and again to the perfectability of the human race through the inheritance of acquired characteristics.[144]

But Condorcet's chief hope for prolongevity was the further progress of medicine. He was too well acquainted with the history and methods of science to limit his horizons to the biological theories current in his own day; in urgent tones, he called on society to organize and support a research program on the most comprehensive scale. Following the lead of Francis Bacon, he sought a planned, systematic investigation of every sort of natural phenomenon; the outline of this scheme was presented in his essay, *On Atlantis*. The medicine of his own day he considered to be still rather ineffectual but on the verge of tremendous progress, because it had learned "to believe nothing but experience."[145] Old age he affirmed to be a natural phenomenon like any other, subject to the laws which rule "organized matter"; as medical research reveals these laws which control the operation of the "human machine" (*cf.* Descartes), physicians will be enabled to keep the body in permanent health, just as a watchmaker by his skill can keep a timepiece in perfect running order.[146]

Malthus attacked all three of the basic assumptions on which Condorcet had built his prolongevitism. First of all, the English theologian denied that the improvement of the environment could bring about any significant increase in longevity; indeed, he doubted that any marked advance could be made in environmental conditions. He expressed scepticism as to whether the masses in any long-settled country could, even in a thousand years, be brought to the level of well-being enjoyed by "the common people, about thirty years ago, in the northern States of America."[147] But even supposing some sort of utopia to be established, with each family in a clean and airy home, both luxury and poverty eliminated and occupational toil and hazards done away with, the result simply would be an enormous increase in population and a return to misery and disease.[148] Condorcet had alluded, in a somewhat veiled manner, to the value of birth control:

. . . even if we agree that the limit [of subsistence] will one day arrive, nothing follows from it that is in the least

188 Antoine-Nicolas de Condorcet, *Fragment sur l'Atlantide, ou efforts combinés de l'espèce humaine pour le progrès des sciences,* in Condorcet, *Œuvres* (see fn. 134) 6: pp. 597–660; this work is hereafter referred to as "Condorcet, *Atlantide.*"
139 Condorcet, *Progress,* p. 199. *Cf.* prolongevity hygiene, see earlier, chap. VII.
140 Condorcet, *Atlantide,* p. 620.
141 On Roger Bacon and the inheritance of acquired characterstics, see earlier, chap. VI.
142 Condorcet, *Progress,* p. 201.

143 *Idem.*
144 Pierre J. G. Cabanis, *Œuvres philosophiques,* Claude Lehec and Jean Cazeneuve, eds., Corpus général des philosophes francais (2 v., Paris, 1956) 1: pp. 160–161, 356–358 and 2: p. 78.
145 Condorcet, *Progress,* p. 158.
146 Condorcet, *Atlantide,* pp. 621–623; *cf.* earlier, Descartes' mechanistic physiology.
147 Malthus, *Essay,* pp. 276–278.
148 *Ibid.,* pp. 181–191.

alarming . . . by then men will know that, if they have a duty towards those who are not yet born, that duty is not to give them existence but to give them happiness; their aim should be to promote the general welfare of the human race . . . rather than foolishly to encumber the world with useless and wretched beings.[149]

But this suggestion was rejected vehemently by Malthus as "unnatural" and, moreover, a threat to "virtue" and "purity of manners." [150]

Malthus also was antipathetic to the other two foundations of Condorcet's optimism: Lamarckism and the progress of medical science. While granting the fact that breeders had been able to effect some improvements in plants and animals, he argued that such advances were far from being without limit.[151] His favorite tactic was to speak of size rather than duration, poking fun at those who might think, for example, of developing a carnation as big as a cabbage or of making potatoes indefinitely large.[152] In regard to the progress of science, Malthus was more circumspect; he admitted that the causes of old age and death were unknown,[153] and that some progress in science might be expected.[154] However, this progress, if any, he felt would be largely in the physical sciences; old age and death he viewed as irremediable concomitants of life.[155] He expressed doubt as to whether in all history there was any example of an increase in the life span, a challenge which still stands today.[156]

CONCLUSION

The most remarkable passage in Malthus' *Essay* is one which, more than a century before Becker, pointed out that the "sceptical" *philosophes* really aimed at a Heavenly City here on earth.

I cannot quit this subject without taking notice of these conjectures of Mr. Godwin and Mr. Condorcet, concerning the indefinite prolongation of human life, as a very curious instance of the longing of the soul after immortality. Both these gentlemen have rejected the light of revelation which absolutely promises eternal life in another state. They have also rejected the light of natural religion, which to the ablest intellects in all ages, has indicated the future existence of the soul. Yet so congenial is the idea of immortality to the mind of man, that they cannot consent entirely to throw it out of their systems. . . . What a strange and curious proof do these conjectures exhibit of the inconsistency of scepticism! [157]

It would be very interesting to know what sort of reply Condorcet would have made to this charge. Actually, it was not until the late nineteenth-century American

physician C. A. Stephens that a prolongevitist dealt with this question in an articulate way; Stephens called his system "natural salvation" and acknowledged that it was patterned on the supernatural salvation of Christianity.[158]

Malthus followed this critique with another noteworthy passage in which he questioned the justice of a progressist solution to the problem of death.

After all their fastidious scepticisms . . . they introduce a species of immortality of their own . . . in the highest degree, narrow, partial and unjust. They suppose all the great, virtuous, and exalted minds, that have ever existed, or that may exist for some thousands, perhaps millions of years, will be sunk in annihilation; and that only a few beings, not greater in number than can exist at once upon the earth, will be ultimately crowned with immortality. Had such a tenet been advanced as a tenet of revelation, I am very sure that all the enemies of religion, and probably Mr. Godwin, and Mr. Condorcet among the rest, would have exhausted the whole force of their ridicule upon it, as the most puerile, the most absurd, the poorest, the most pitiful, the most iniquitously unjust, and, consequently, the most unworthy of the Deity, that the superstitious folly of man could invent.

The point still is being echoed by twentieth-century proponents of neo-orthodoxy, who argue that, for a just solution of the problem of death, all generations must be equal.[159] To be sure, neither Condorcet nor Godwin made any claim of being able to replace all the promises of traditional religion with equivalent ones based on science and progress. Nevertheless, the logic of their position would seem to drive them towards an acknowledgment of the desirability of resurrection. And in view of their faith in the unlimited perfectability of man and the immeasurable advance of science, it would seem that they might have speculated on its possibility as well.[160]

---

[149] Condorcet, *Progress*, pp. 188–189.

[150] Malthus, *Essay*, p. 154.

[151] *Ibid.*, pp. 163–167.

[152] *Ibid.*, pp. 166, 249.

[153] *Ibid.*, p. 168.

[154] *Ibid.*, p. 232.

[155] *Ibid.*, pp. 239–240.

[156] *Ibid.*, pp. 157–158, 160–161. On "life span" and "life expectancy," see earlier, chap. I.

[157] *Ibid.*, pp. 240–242.

[158] C. A. Stephens, *Natural Salvation: the Message of Science* (Norway Lake, Maine, 1903). *Cf.*, by the present author, "C. A. Stephens—Popular Author and Prophet of Gerontology," *New England Journal of Medicine* 254 (1956): pp. 658–660 and "C. A. Stephens—a Pioneer of American Gerontology," *Geriatrics* 14 (1959): pp. 332–336. Stephens and other Darwinists will be discussed in my work, *Death and Progress: the Rise of Secular Salvation*.

[159] Nicholas Berdyaev, *The Meaning of History* (London, 1936), pp. 189 ff. and John Baillie, *The Belief in Progress* (London, 1950), pp. 183–185. The dictum that "all generations are equal" also is central in Ranke's "historicism"; Pieter Geyl, *Debates with Historians* (Cleveland and New York, 1958), pp. 9–29.

[160] At least one nineteenth-century thinker carried the idea of progress this far. On Nicholas Fedorov, see James H. Billington, "The Intelligentsia and the Religion of Humanity," *Amer. Hist. Review* 65 (1960): pp. 813–814 and Jacques Choron, *Modern Man and Mortality* (New York, 1964), pp. 11–12. More information on Fedorov is found in Nicholas Berdyaev, *The Russian Idea* (Boston, 1962), pp. 208–212; and V. V. Zenkovsky, *A History of Russian Philosophy*, George L. Kline, transl. (2 v., New York and London, 1953) 2: pp. 588–604. Berdyaev states that Fedorov had a profound effect on Tolstoy, Dostoyevsky, Solovev, and Berdyaev himself. A more mystical solution to the ethical problem of progress was provided by Pierre Leroux in his doctrine of palingenesis; see Bury, *op. cit.* (see fn. 2), pp. 318–320; and D. G. Charlton,

In conclusion, it should be noted that Condorcet, through his disciple Cabanis, had a marked influence in initiating the golden age of French medicine. The *philosophe* had that dual personality so characteristic of many of the greatest scientists: an almost religious zeal and enthusiasm combined with a high standard of intellectual honesty; in the words of a contemporary, he was "a volcano covered with snow." [161] He had done valuable scientific work himself, especially in mathematics, and for long he was secretary of the Academy of Sciences [162]; hence it is not surprising that he was an advocate of the most sophisticated methodology including symbolic logic and the statistics of probability. [163] This unusual combination of ardent optimism and cool-headed objectivity was passed on to his follower, Cabanis. And Cabanis was a dominant figure in founding the "Paris school" which rejected the dogmatic systems of eighteenth-century medicine and built up instead a routine of medical practice based directly on observations made in the clinic and at autopsies. [164] During the first half of the nineteenth century, French medicine led the world.

IX. EPILOGUE

Condorcet, Franklin, and other eighteenth-century savants envisaged the indefinite prolongation of life as a goal of science; but it has been often pointed out that recent achievements have not extended the maximum (and presumably biologic) limits of the life span. If the day ever does come when a much higher expectancy is attained, the most momentous results would obviously follow. The future of society would then turn in no small degree on developments in medicine, much as the outcome in medicine has always depended in part upon trends within society.
R. H. Shryock, "The Significance of Medicine in American History," 1956 [1]

One can speak of the evolution of the idea of prolongevity as separable into two large segments, with the Enlightenment serving as the point of division. The earlier part would range from the beginnings of human culture down into the eighteenth century; the other would cover developments from that time on to the present. The reasons for choosing the Enlightenment period as a turning point are that the idea of progress (replacing primitivism) provides a new ideological basis for prolongevitism, and the scientific revolution of the sixteenth and seventeenth centuries heralds the ending of proto-science and the beginning of a scientific foundation for prolongevitism.

In this study, we have dealt with the main currents of prolongevity thought before 1800, attempting to show that there is more substance and timeliness to this "early" history than generally is recognized. It is customary in scholarly and professional writings, as well as popular ones, to handle the beginnings of prolongevity in a rather slighting way. The merest mention of Methuselah, the fountain of youth, the alchemist's elixir, and, sometimes, a more respectful nod in the direction of Francis Bacon—these are considered to cover the subject sufficiently. Indeed, that was the view of the present author when he undertook this work: a single chapter was thought to be ample for the material studied here. However, it soon became evident that an entire monograph might be desirable in order to do justice to the various strands in "early" prolongevitism.

We have seen, for example, that the idea of prolongevity is not a simple one, comprising, as it does, a variety of goals to be aimed at and methods to be employed; and it was shown that the concepts of life expectancy and life span must be differentiated with care. The forces (apologism) arraigned against prolongevity were found to hold strong positions in legend and folklore, in philosophy, in science and medicine, and in religion. Despite the power of apologism, however, prolongevity folklore has been seen as virtually ubiquitous, its three chief variants (antediluvian, hyperborean, and fountain themes) appearing in almost all cultures, at nearly every period of history.

Further, we have learned that, regardless of certain apologist tendencies in Taoist thought, the classics did provide a respectable intellectual framework for a systematic prolongevitism—the first in history. And Taoist physiological practices were demonstrated to be related to an accumulation of genuine (though often misinterpreted) empirical observations. The same may be said for Chinese alchemy, especially in connection with the remarkable chemical behavior of mercury and its compounds. We have examined also the prolongevity rationale worked out for Latin alchemy by Roger Bacon and have traced the rise of the Lullian school, with its search for a "quintessence" and its contribution to the iatrochemistry of Paracelsus. A problem for comparative history was posed by the lack of direct evidence that Arabic alchemy served as a bridge between East and West.

It has been noted that Cornaro's *Discorsi* correlates well with the Burckhardtian theory of the Renaissance and begins a tradition of prolongevity hygiene carried, via Lessius, Hufeland, and others, to the end of the nine-

---

Secular Religions in France: 1815–1870 (London and New York, 1963), pp. 82–87. These matters are discussed in detail in my work *Death and Progress: the Rise of Secular Salvation.* Meanwhile, it must be reported that in one of C. A. Stephens' notebooks, in the collection of this author, there appears the following memo: "Have your own body embalmed at your death in hope that ere many decades death will be vanquished and the resurrection be brought within scientific possibilities. It will stand as a proof of your sincerity and help propagate the Great Truth."

[161] Schapiro, *op. cit.* (see fn. 134), p. 77.
[162] *Ibid.*, pp. 67–69.
[163] Condorcet, *Progress*, pp. 190–191, 197–199.
[164] Erwin H. Ackerknecht, *A Short History of Medicine* (New York, 1955), p. 135.
[1] Richard H. Shryock, "The Significance of Medicine in American History," *Amer. Historical Review* 62 (1956): pp. 81–91; 91. See also, the same author's *The Development of Modern Medicine* (Philadelphia and London, 1936), pp. 76–77, 419–423.

teenth century. Carl Becker's thesis on the "uses of posterity" was scrutinized and found helpful in explaining the prolongevity trend among the *philosophes*—Descartes, Bacon, Franklin, Godwin, and Condorcet;[2] also it was seen that Malthus anticipated the Becker theme and projected arguments still viable in the clash between neo-orthodoxy and "natural salvation." Moreover, Enlightenment prolongevitism was shown to have influenced the beginnings of experimental physiology, blood transfusion, resuscitation, and anabiosis.

Having reviewed some of the main points of the monograph, it might be well to recall three of the aims stated in the first chapter: (1) The evolution of ideas about the prolongation of life has been long and complex and elucidates significant areas in the history of ideas. (2) The chief prolongevity hypotheses were reasonable deductions from major scientific and philosophical currents of their time. (3) Belief in the possibility and desirability of prolongevity furthered the progress of science and medicine. Hopefully, these proposals have been exemplified sufficiently in the text to make further repetition of the data unnecessary at this point.

It may be of interest here to give a very brief survey of certain outstanding trends in the history of prolongevity since about 1800.[3] The influence of the Enlightenment continued in three of the strongest currents of thought in the nineteenth century. First, utopianism: most, but not all, utopian schemes promised some increase in the length of healthy life. Second, Darwinism: although there were apologist Darwinists (e.g., Weismann), others were firmly prolongevitist, as, for example, Metchnikoff, Winwood Reade, and C. A. Stephens (*Natural Salvation*). Third, Marxism: prolongevity has been a recurrent theme (along with some glimmerings of apologism) in Marxist writings and persists to the present, not only in orthodox communist circles but also among many social democrats, as well as some Christian socialists and eclectic liberals.

About the beginning of the twentieth century, there was a marked change in the character of prolongevity concepts, as the aging population and the welfare state in industrially advanced societies brought a concern with senescence less dependent on ideological considerations. Gerontology has become a recognized specialty, and increasing sums are being expended by foundations and governments in research on aging. Along with the growth of gerontology, there have come a number of bio-medical observations which offer some hope to prolongevitists: e.g., the effect of sex hormones on such conditions as osteoporosis and skin atrophy, the "im-mortality" of tissue cultures, the relation between diet and atherosclerosis, the prolongation of life in various species by underfeeding, the protective action of glycerol in the freezing of mammalian cells, and the isolation of a "status quo" hormone in insects and, perhaps, in some mammals.

With these encouraging twentieth-century occurrences have come some contrary trends. The social and economic upheavals of this century have placed very much in doubt the sort of idea of progress held in the previous century. Not that meliorism has been abandoned; on the contrary, the "revolution of rising expectations" indicates how deeply modern culture is committed to a progressist view. But, along with this, there has been a sharp counter-revolution of falling expectations, and the contemporary mind is torn by deep contradictions. Small wonder that this is an era characterized by inner conflict and anxiety. There is a pervasive fear that life is meaningless, absurd; and the dilemma weighs most heavily on the individual and his debatable "worth."

As stated in the first pages of this study, the present author feels that in the crisis of our time, the best course would be a conscious furthering of the meliorist tradition, and, in regard to the problem of death, the forwarding of efforts for prolongevity. This means that a program of action would be supported to augment, in tangible ways, the value of each person: through prolongevity, rejuvenation, resuscitation techniques, and, perhaps, even some variety of resurrection. The "worth" of the individual is, one might suggest, not so much a fact as a goal.

BIBLIOGRAPHY

I. a. History of Gerontology and Geriatrics

BURSTEIN, SONA ROSA. 1946. "Gerontology: a Modern Science with a Long History." *Post Graduate Medical Journal* (London) **22**: pp. 185–190.

—— 1955, 1957. "The Historical Background of Gerontology." *Geriatrics* **10**: pp. 189–193, 328–332, 536–540 and **12**: pp. 494–499.

FREEMAN, JOSEPH T. 1938. "The History of Geriatrics." *Annals of Medical History* **10**: pp. 324–335.

—— 1961. "Nascher: Excerpts from his Life, Letters, and Works." *The Gerontologist* **1**: pp. 17–26.

FREEMAN, JOSEPH T., and IRVING L. WEBBER, eds. 1965. *Perspectives in Aging.* Supplement to *The Gerontologist* **5**, 1: Part 2.

GRMEK, MIRKO D. 1958. "On Ageing and Old Age: Basic Problems and Historic Aspects of Gerontology and Geriatrics." *Monographiae biologicae* **5**, 2 (Den Haag).

GRUMAN, GERALD J. 1957. "An Introduction to Literature on the History of Gerontology." *Bull. Hist. of Medicine* **31**: pp. 78–83.

PHILIBERT, MICHEL. 1964. *The Development of Social Gerontology in the U.S.A.* (mimeo., Ann Arbor).

SHOCK, NATHAN W., ed. 1951, 1957, 1963. *A Classified Bibliography of Gerontology and Geriatrics* (Stanford, Calif.). *Supplement One: 1949–1955. Supplement Two: 1956–1961.*

STEUDEL, JOHANNES. 1942. "Zur Geschichte der Lehre von den Greisenkrankheiten." *Sudhoffs Archiv für Geschichte der Medizin und der Naturwissenschaften* **35**: pp. 1–27.

---

[2] The term *philosophe* is used here in a general sense to include Descartes, Bacon, and Godwin.

[3] The period after 1800 will be covered in some detail, but from a rather broader point of view, in my work *Death and Progress: the Rise of Secular Salvation.*

ZEMAN, FREDERIC D. 1942–1950. "Life's Later Years: Studies in the Medical History of Old Age." *Jour. Mt. Sinai Hospital* (N. Y.) **8**: pp. 1161–1165; **11**: pp. 45–52, 97–104, 224–231, 300–307, 339–344; **12**: pp. 783–791, 833–846, 890–901, 939–953; **13**: pp. 241–256; **16**: pp. 308–322; and **17**: pp. 53–68.

I. b. *Other Works*

CALDER, NIGEL, ed. 1965. *The World in 1984* (2 v., Baltimore and Harmondsworth) 2.
CASTIGLIONI, ARTURO. 1947. *A History of Medicine*, E. B. Krumbhaar, tr. and ed. (2nd ed., New York).
CHAMBERS, CLARKE A. 1958. "The Belief in Progress in Twentieth-Century America." *Jour. Hist. of Ideas* **19**: pp. 197–224.
CHORON, JACQUES. 1963. *Death and Western Thought* (New York and London).
—— 1964. *Modern Man and Mortality* (New York).
COMFORT, ALEX. 1964. *Ageing: the Biology of Senescence* (2nd ed., New York).
—— 1964. *The Process of Ageing,* Signet Science Library (New York).
DUBLIN, LOUIS I. 1957. "Outlook for Longevity in the United States." *Newsletter Gerontological Society* **4**, 2: p. 3.
DUBLIN, LOUIS I., A. J. LOTKA and M. SPIEGELMAN. 1949. *Length of Life: a Study of the Life Table* (rev. ed., New York).
FEIFEL, HERMAN, ed. 1959. *The Meaning of Death* (New York).
FULTON, ROBERT, ed. 1965. *Death and Identity* (New York, London, Sydney).
GINSBERG, MORRIS. 1953. *The Idea of Progress: a Revaluation* (Boston).
HOFFMAN, FREDERICK J. 1964. *The Mortal No: Death and the Modern Imagination* (Princeton).
IGGERS, GEORG G. 1965. "The Idea of Progress: a Critical Reassessment," *Amer. Hist. Review* **71**: pp. 1–17.
LANSING, ALBERT I., ed. 1952. *Cowdry's Problems of Ageing: Biological and Medical Aspects* (3rd ed., Baltimore).
SHOCK, NATHAN W. 1957. *Trends in Gerontology* (2nd ed., Stanford, Calif.).
VOGT, EVON Z., and JOHN M. ROBERTS. 1956. "A Study of Values." *Scientific American* **195**, 1: pp. 25–30.
WILES, PETER. 1965. "On Physical Immortality," *Survey* (London) 56, pp. 125–143; 57, pp. 142–161.

II. a. *Apologism: Primary Sources*

(ARISTOTLE). Ross, W. D., and J. A. Smith, eds. 1908–1952. *The Works of Aristotle, Translated into English* (12 v., Oxford).
(AUGUSTINE). Dods, Marcus, tr. 1950. *The City of God,* Modern Library (New York).
AVICENNA. *Canon of Medicine,* book one. In Gruner. 1930. See II. b.
(CICERO). Peabody, Andrew P., tr. 1887. *De senectute* (Boston).
(GALEN). Brock, Arthur J., tr. 1916. *On the Natural Faculties,* Loeb Classical Library (London and New York).
(——). Green, Robert Montraville, tr. 1951. *Galen's Hygiene: De sanitate tuenda* (Springfield, Ill.).
(GALEN, and others). Brock, Arthur J., ed. 1929. *Greek Medicine: Being Extracts Illustrative of Medical Writers from Hippocrates to Galen,* Library of Greek Thought (London, Toronto and New York).
(Gilgamesh Epic). In Heidel. 1949. See II. b.
(——). Sandars, N. K., ed. 1960. *The Epic of Gilgamesh* (Baltimore).
(HESIOD). Brown, Norman O., tr. 1953. *Hesiod's Theogony,* Library of Liberal Arts 36 (New York).

(——). Evelyn-White, Hugh G., tr. 1914. *Hesiod, the Homeric Hymns and Homerica,* Loeb Classical Library (London and New York).
(HIPPOCRATES). Jones, W. H. S., and E. T. Withington, tr. 1923–1931. *Hippocrates,* Loeb Classical Library (4 v., London and New York).
(JUVENAL). Ramsay, G. G., tr. 1950. "Satires," in *Juvenal and Persius,* Loeb Classical Library (Cambridge, Mass. and London), pp. 3–307.
(LUCRETIUS). Latham, Ronald E., tr. 1951. *Lucretius, On the Nature of the Universe* (Harmondsworth, Middlesex).
(MARCUS AURELIUS). Jackson, John, tr. 1948. *The Thoughts of Marcus Aurelius Antoninus,* The World's Classics (London).
(Myths). Henderson, Joseph L., and Maud Oakes, eds. 1963. See II. b.
(New Testament). Revised Standard Version. 1946. *The New Testament* (Toronto, New York, and Edinburgh).
(Old Testament). Revised Standard Version. 1952. *The Old Testament* (2 v., Toronto, New York, and Edinburgh).
(SOPHOCLES). Storr, F., tr. 1924. *Sophocles,* Loeb Classical Library (2 v., London).
(Stoics and Epicureans). Oates, Whitney J., ed. 1940. *The Stoic and Epicurean Philosophers: the Complete Extant Writings of Epicurus, Epictetus, Lucretius and Marcus Aurelius* (New York).
(THOMAS AQUINAS). Fathers of the English Dominican Province, tr. 1912–1922. *Summa theologica* (20 v., London).

II. b. *Apologism: Secondary Works*

ALEXANDER, I. E., R. S. COLLEY and A. M. ADLERSTEIN. 1957. "Is Death a Matter of Indifference?" *Jour. Psychology* **43**: pp. 277–283.
BECKER, CARL L. 1932. See VIII. b.
BEWER, JULIUS A. 1933. *The Literature of the Old Testament* (New York).
BURY, J. B. 1932. See VIII. b.
CHORON, JACQUES. 1963. See I. b.
CLARKE, M. L. 1956. *The Roman Mind: Studies in the History of Thought from Cicero to Marcus Aurelius* (London).
DE WITT, NORMAN WENTWORTH. 1954. *Epicurus and his Philosophy* (Minneapolis).
FESTINGER, LEON. 1962. "Cognitive Dissonance." *Scientific American* **207**, 4: pp. 93–102.
FRAZER, JAMES G. 1918. *Folk-Lore in the Old Testament* (3 v., London).
GRUNER, O. C. 1930. *A Treatise on the Canon of Medicine of Avicenna, Incorporating a Translation of the First Book* (London).
HEIDEL, ALEXANDER. 1949. *The Gilgamesh Epic and Old Testament Parallels* (2nd ed., Chicago).
HENDERSON, JOSEPH L., and MAUD OAKES, eds. 1963. *The Wisdom of the Serpent: the Myths of Death, Rebirth, and Resurrection* (New York).
KALISH, RICHARD A. 1966. "A Continuum of Subjectively Perceived Death." *The Gerontologist* **6**: pp. 73–76.
KRAMER, SAMUEL NOAH. 1956. *From the Tablets of Sumer* (Indian Hills, Colorado).
SARTON, GEORGE. 1954. *Galen of Pergamon,* Logan Clendening Lectures on the History and Philosophy of Medicine **3** (Lawrence, Kansas).
SHEPS, JACK. 1957. "Management of Fear of Death in Chronic Disease." *Jour. Amer. Geriatrics Society* **5**: pp. 793–797.
SINGER, CHARLES. 1950. *A History of Biology* (rev. ed., New York).
SOLMSEN, FRIEDRICH. 1949. *Hesiod and Aeschylus,* Cornell Studies in Classical Philology **30** (Ithaca, N. Y.).

WESTERMANN, WILLIAM L. 1955. *The Slave Systems of Greek and Roman Antiquity*, Mem. Amer. Philos. Soc. **40** (Philadelphia).

WICKENS, G. M., ed. 1952. *Avicenna, Scientist and Philosopher: a Millenary Symposium* (London).

ZELLER, EDUARD. 1880. *The Stoics, Epicureans and Sceptics* (London).

—— 1931. *Outlines of the History of Greek Philosophy*, International Library of Psychology, Philosophy and Scientific Method (13th ed., London and New York).

ZINKER, JOSEPH C., and STEPHEN L. FINK. 1966. "The Possibility for Psychological Growth in a Dying Person." *Jour. General Psychology* **74**: pp. 185–199.

III a. *Prolongevity Legends: Primary Sources*

(Alexander Legends). Budge, E. A. Wallis, tr. 1896. *The Life and Exploits of Alexander the Great, Being a Series of Translations of the Ethiopic Histories of Alexander* (London).

(——). In Meyer, Paul. 1886. See III. *b.*

(Apocrypha). Charles, Robert H., ed. 1913. *Apocrypha and Pseudepigrapha of the Old Testament* (2 v., Oxford).

(AUGUSTINE). 1950. See II. *a.*

(BACON, ROGER). 1923. See VI. *a.*

(Bran, Voyage of). In Meyer and Nutt. 1895. See III. *b.*

(FONTANEDA, HERNANDO D'ESCALENTE). Smith, Buckingham, tr. 1944. *Memoir* (Miami, Fla.).

(GRIMM, JAKOB L. K., and WILHELM K. GRIMM). Scharl, Joseph, ed. 1948. *Grimm's Fairy Tales* (London).

(HERODOTUS). Godley, A. D., tr. 1921. *Herodotus*, Loeb Classical Library (4 v., London).

(JOSEPHUS). Thackeray, H. St. J., and Ralph Marcus, tr. 1930.ᐧ *Josephus*, Loeb Classical Library (9 v., London and New York).

(Koran). Pickthall, Mohammed Marmaduke, tr. and ed. 1953. *The Meaning of the Glorious Koran: an Explanatory Translation* (New York).

(MANDEVILLE, SIR JOHN). 1915. *Travels*, Library of English Classics (London).

(Old Testament). 1952. See II. *a.*

(OVID). Miller, Frank Justus, tr. 1916. *Metamorphoses*, Loeb Classical Library (2 v., London and New York).

(PAUSANIAS). Jones, W. H. S., tr. 1918. *Description of Greece*, Loeb Classical Library (6 v., London and New York).

(PETER MARTYR D'ANGHIERA). MacNutt, Francis A., tr. 1912. *De orbe novo* (2 v., New York).

(PINDAR). Sandys, Sir John, tr. 1919. *Pindar*, Loeb Classical Library (London and New York).

(PLINY). Bostock, John, and H. T. Riley, tr. 1855 ff. *Natural History* (6 v., London).

(PLUTARCH). Perrin, Bernadotte, tr. 1919. *Plutarch's Lives*, Loeb Classical Library (11 v., London and New York).

(STRABO). JONES, HORACE L., tr. 1917. *Geography*, Loeb Classical Library (8 v., London and New York).

(VERGIL). Mackail, J. W., tr. 1950. *Virgil's Works*, Modern Library (New York).

III. b. *Prolongevity Legends: Secondary Works*

ABEL, ARMAND. 1955. *Le Roman d'Alexandre*, Collections Lebeque et nationale **112** (Brussels).

BARRAUD, GEORGES. 1952. "De la Fontaine de jouvence aux cures thermales chez les anciens." *Bull. médical* (Paris) **66**: pp. 361–362.

BEAUVOIS, EUG. 1884. "La Fontaine de jouvence et le Jourdain dans les traditions des Antilles et de la Floride." *Le Muséon* (Louvain) **3**: pp. 404–429.

BENEDICT, RUTH. 1933. "Magic." *Encyclopedia of the Social Sciences* (New York) **10**: pp. 39–44.

BETHUNE-BAKER, J. F. 1933. *Introduction to the Early History of Christian Doctrine* (5th ed., London).

VAN DEN BIESEN, C. 1907–1914. "Antediluvians." *Catholic Encyclopedia* (New York) **1**: pp. 551–553.

BOAS, GEORGE. 1948. *Essays on Primitivism and Related Ideas in the Middle Ages* (Baltimore).

COMFORT, ALEX. 1961. "The Life Span of Animals." *Scientific American* **205**, 2: pp. 108–119.

DAWSON, W. R. 1929. *Magician and Leech* (London).

ETTINGER, ROBERT C. W. 1964. 1965. 1966. See VIII. *b.*

FRAZER, JAMES G. 1900. *The Golden Bough: a Study in Magic and Religion* (12 v., London).

HAMILTON, EDITH. 1953. *Mythology* (New York).

HARRISON, THOMAS P. 1960. "Bird of Paradise: Phoenix Redivivus." *Isis* **51**: pp. 173–180.

HASTINGS, JAMES, ed. 1908–1922. *Encyclopedia of Religion and Ethics* (12 v., New York).

HOPKINS, EDWARD WASHBURN. 1905. "The Fountain of Youth." *Jour. Amer. Oriental Society* **26**: pp. 1–67.

LAWSON, EDWARD W. 1946. *The Discovery of Florida and its Discoverer Juan Ponce de León* (St. Augustine, Fla.).

(Life Extension Society). 1964 ff. See VIII. *b.*

LOVEJOY, ARTHUR O., and GEORGE BOAS. 1935. *Primitivism and Related Ideas in Antiquity* (Baltimore).

MASSON, LOUIS. 1937, 1938. "La Fontaine de jouvence." *Aesculape* (Paris) **27**: pp. 244–251 and **28**: pp. 16–23.

MCCARTNEY, EUGENE S. 1925. "Longevity and Rejuvenation in Greek and Roman Folklore." *Papers Michigan Acad. of Science, Arts and Letters* **5**: pp. 37–72.

MEYER, KUNO, and ALFRED NUTT. 1895. *The Voyage of Bran, Son of Febal, to the Land of the Living*, Grimm Library **4** (London).

MEYER, PAUL. 1886. *Alexandre le Grand dans la littérature française du moyen âge*, Bibliothèque française du moyen âge (2 v., Paris).

MORISON, SAMUEL ELIOT. 1942. *Admiral of the Ocean Sea; a Life of Christopher Columbus* (Boston).

PARKES, A. S. 1955. See VIII. *b.*

RICHARDSON, BESSIE ELLEN. 1933. *Old Age among the Ancient Greeks* (Baltimore).

RIVERS, W. H. R. 1924. *Medicine, Magic and Religion*, International Library of Psychology, Philosophy and Scientific Method (London and New York).

SIMMONS, LEO W. 1945. *The Role of the Aged in Primitive Society* (New Haven).

SPENCE, LEWIS. 1913. *A Dictionary of Medieval Romance and Romance Writers* (London and New York).

TALBOT, CHARLES. 1957. "The Fountain of Life: a Greek Version." *Bull. Hist. of Medicine* **31**: pp. 1–16.

THOMPSON, STITH. 1955–1958. *Motif-Index of Folk-Literature* (6 v., rev. ed., Bloomington, Ind.).

UNDERHILL, EVELYN. 1910. "The Fountain of Life: an Iconographical Study." *Burlington Magazine* **17**: pp. 99–109.

IV. and V. a. *The Taoists: Primary Sources*

(CHUANG TZU). Legge, James, tr. 1891. *Chuang Tzu*. In *The Texts of Taoism*, Sacred Books of the East (2 v., Oxford) **1**: pp. 127–392 and **2**: pp. 1–232.

(*Hsien* literature). Giles, Lionel, tr. 1948. *A Gallery of Chinese Immortals*, Wisdom of the East (London).

Ko HUNG. *Pao-p'u Tzu*. See VI. *a.*

(LAO TZU). Balfour, Frederic Henry, tr. 1884. *Tao Te Ching*. In *Taoist Texts: Ethical, Political and Speculative* (London and Shanghai), pp. 1–48.

(——). Legge, James, tr. 1891. *Tao Te Ching*. In *The Texts of Taoism*, Sacred Books of the East (2 v., Oxford) **1**: pp. 45–124.

——*Tao Te Ching*. In Waley. 1935; 1958. See IV. and V. *b.*

(LIEH TZU). Giles, Lionel, tr. 1912. *Taoist Teachings from the Book of Lieh Tzu,* Wisdom of the East (London).

(——). Wieger, Léon, tr. 1913; 1953. *Les Pères du système taoiste* (Hsienhsien; Paris), pp. 65–199.

(——). Wilhelm, Richard, tr. 1921. *Liä Dsi* (Jena).

(Nine Songs). Waley, Arthur, tr. and ed. 1955. *The Nine Songs: a Study of Shamanism in Ancient China* (London).

IV. and V. *b. The Taoists: Secondary Works*

(See also, the works on Chinese alchemy in list VI.)

AMIOT, J. J. M. 1779. "Notice du cong-fou." *Mémoires concernant l'histoire, les sciences, etc. des Chinois; par les missionnaires de Pe-kin* (Paris) **4**: pp. 441–451.

CHAN, WING-TSIT. 1953. *Religious Trends in Modern China* (New York).

DUBS, HOMER H. 1946. "Taoism." In *China,* Harley F. MacNair, ed., United Nations Series (Berkeley, Calif.), pp. 266–289.

DUDGEON, JOHN. 1895. "Kung-fu, or Medical Gymnastics." *Jour. Peking Oriental Society* **3**: pp. 341–565.

DUYVENDAK, J. J. L. 1934. "Taoism." In *Encyclopedia of the Social Sciences* (New York) **14**: pp. 510–513.

ELIADE, MIRCEA. 1951. *Le Chamanisme* (Paris).

FUNG YU-LAN. 1952. *History of Chinese Philosophy,* Derk Bodde, tr. (2 v., Princeton).

GILES, HERBERT A. 1898. *A Chinese Biographical Dictionary* (London and Shanghai).

DE GROOT, J. J. M. 1910. *The Religion of the Chinese* (New York).

MASPERO, HENRI. 1937. "Les Procédés de 'nourrir le principe vital' dans la religion taoiste ancienne." *Jour. asiatique* **229**: pp. 177–252, 353–430.

—— 1950. *Le Taoisme* (Paris).

MASPERO, HENRI, and JEAN ESCARRA. 1952. *Les Institutions de la Chine* (Paris).

MORSE, W. R. 1934. *Chinese Medicine* (New York).

NEEDHAM, JOSEPH. 1954 ff. *Science and Civilization in China* (Cambridge).

PEILLON, MARCELLE. 1948. "Gymnastique et massages." In *Histoire générale de la médecine,* M. Laignel-Lavastine, ed. (Paris) **3**: pp. 627–642.

WALEY, ARTHUR. 1935; 1958. *The Way and its Power: a Study of the Tao Te Ching and its Place in Chinese Thought* (Boston; New York).

WEBER, MAX. 1951. *The Religion of China: Confucianism and Taoism,* Hans H. Gerth, tr. (Glenco, Ill.).

WEI, FRANCIS C. M. 1947. *The Spirit of Chinese Culture* (New York).

WELCH, HOLMES. 1956. "Syncretism in the Early Taoist Movement." *Papers on China,* East Asia Program, Committee on Regional Studies, Harvard University (Cambridge, Mass.) **10**: pp. 1–54.

—— 1957. *The Parting of the Way: Lao Tzu and the Taoist Movement* (Boston).

WERNER, E. T. C. 1932. *A Dictionary of Chinese Mythology* (Shanghai).

WIEGER, LÉON. 1913; 1953. *Le Canon taoiste* (Hsienhsien; Paris).

YÜ, YING-SHIH. 1964–1965. "Life and Immortality in the Mind of Han China." *Harvard Jour. Asiatic Studies* **25**: pp. 80–122.

VI. *a. The Alchemists: Primary Sources*

(Arabic alchemists). Berthelot, Marcellin, ed. 1893. *L'Alchimie arabe.* In *Histoire des sciences: la chimie au moyen âge* (3 v., Paris) **3**.

(ARNALD OF VILLANOVA). Sigerist, Henry E., tr. and ed. 1943. *The Earliest Printed Book on Wine* (New York).

(AVICENNA). Holmyard, E. J., and D. C. Mandeville, tr. 1927. *Avicennae De congelatione et conglutinatione lapidum* (Paris).

(BACON, ROGER). Browne, Richard, tr. 1683. *Cure of Old Age, and Preservation of Youth* (London).

(——). Burke, Robert Belle, tr. 1928. *Opus majus* (2 v., Philadelphia and London).

(——). Davis, Tenney L., tr. 1923. *Letter Concerning the Marvelous Power of Art and of Nature* (Easton, Pa., London, and Tokyo).

(——). Little, A. G., and E. Withington, eds. 1928. *De retardatione accidentium senectutis, cum aliis opusculis de rebus medicinalibus,* British Society of Franciscan Studies **14** (Oxford).

(DASTIN, JOHN). Josten, C. H., tr. 1949. "Letter to Pope John XXII." *Ambix* **4**: pp. 34–51.

(GEBER). Darmstaedter, Ernst, tr. and ed. 1922. *Die Alchemie des Geber* (Berlin).

(——). Russell, Richard, tr., and E. J. Holmyard, ed. 1928. *Works* (London and New York).

(Hellenistic alchemists). Berthelot, Marcellin, tr. 1888. *Collection des anciens alchimistes grecs* (3 v., Paris).

(IBN KHALDUN). Rosenthal, Franz, tr. 1958. *The Muqaddimah: an Introduction to History,* Bollingen Series **43** (3 v., New York).

(AL-IRAQI, ABU'L-QASIM). Holmyard, E. J., tr. 1923. *Book of Knowledge Acquired Concerning the Cultivation of Gold,* Librairie orientaliste (Paris).

(Ko HUNG). Ch'en Kuo-fu, and Tenney L. Davis, tr. 1941. *Pao-p'u Tzu,* chapters 8 and 11, and summaries of the others. *Proceedings Amer. Acad. of Arts and Sciences* **74**: pp. 297–325.

(——). Davis, Tenney L., and Lu-ch'iang Wu, tr. 1935. *Pao-p'u Tzu,* chapters 4 and 16. *Proceedings Amer. Acad. of Arts and Sciences* **70**: pp. 221–284.

(——). Feifel, Eugene, tr. 1941–1946. *Pao-p'u Tzu,* chapters 1, 2, 3, 4, and 11. *Monumenta Serica* (Peking) **6**: pp. 113–211, **9**: pp. 1–33, and **11**: pp. 1–32.

(PARACELSUS). Waite, Arthur Edward, tr. 1894. *The Hermetic and Alchemical Writings of Paracelsus* (2 v., London).

(AL-RAZI). Ruska, Julius, tr. 1937. *Al-Razi's Buch Geheimnis der Geheimnisse,* Quellen und Studien zur Geschichte der Naturwissenschaften und der Medizin **6** (Berlin).

(STEPHANOS OF ALEXANDRIA). Taylor, F. Sherwood, tr. 1937–1938. "The Alchemical Works of Stephanos of Alexandria." *Ambix* **1**: pp. 116–139 and **2**: pp. 39–49.

(Syriac alchemists). Berthelot, Marcellin, ed. 1893. *L'Alchimie syriaque.* In *Histoire des sciences: la chimie au moyen âge* (3 v., Paris) **2**.

(WEI PO-YANG). Wu, Lu-ch'iang, and Tenney L. Davis, tr. 1932. *Ts'an T'ung Ch'i.* In *Isis* **18**: pp. 210–289.

VI. *b. The Alchemists: Secondary Works*

AHMAD, MAQBUL, and B. B. DATTA. 1929. "A Persian Translation of the Eleventh Century Arabic Alchemical Treatise *Ain As-San'ah Wa 'Aun As-Sana'ah.*" *Memoirs Asiatic Society of Bengal* (Calcutta) **8**: pp. 419–460.

"Alchemy." 1957. *Encyclopedia of Chemistry,* George L. Clark, ed. (New York), pp. 28–29.

'ALI, M. TURAB, H. E. STAPLETON and M. HIDAYAT HUSAIN. 1933. "Three Arabic Treatises on Alchemy by Muhammad Bin Umail." *Memoirs Asiatic Society of Bengal* (Calcutta) **12**: pp. 1–213.

ALLENDY, R. 1912. *L'Alchimie et la médecine: études sur les théories hermétiques dans l'histoire de la médecine* (Paris).

AMADOU, ROBERT. 1953. *Raymond Lulle et l'alchimie* (Paris?).

BERTHELOT, MARCELLIN. 1885. *Les Origines de l'alchimie* (Paris).
—— 1938. *Introduction à l'étude de la chimie des anciens et du moyen-âge* (Paris).
BRIDGES, JOHN HENRY. 1914. *The Life and Work of Roger Bacon* (London).
CHIKASHIGE, MASUMI. 1936. *Alchemy and Other Chemical Achievements of the Ancient Orient* (Tokyo).
COHEN, I. BERNARD. 1951. "Ethan Allen Hitchcock: Soldier, Humanitarian, Scholar—Discoverer of the 'True Subject' of the Hermetic Art." *Proceedings Amer. Antiquarian Society* 61: pp. 29–136.
CROMBIE, A. C. 1959. *Medieval and Early Modern Science* (2nd ed., 2 v., Garden City, N. Y.).
DAVIS, TENNEY L. 1936. "The Problem of the Origins of Alchemy." *Scientific Monthly* 43: pp. 551–558.
—— 1943. "The Chinese Beginnings of Alchemy." *Endeavor* 2: pp. 154–160.
DAVIS, TENNEY L., and LU-CH'IANG WU. 1930. "Chinese Alchemy." *Scientific Monthly* 31: pp. 225–235.
DEBUS, ALLEN G. 1962. "An Elizabethan History of Medical Chemistry." *Annals of Science* 18: pp. 1–29.
—— 1964. See VIII. *b.*
—— 1964. "Robert Fludd and the Use of Gilbert's *De Magnete* in the Weapon-Salve Controversy." *Jour. Hist. Medicine and Allied Sciences* 19: pp. 389–417.
—— 1965. *The English Paracelsians* (London).
—— 1965. "The Significance of the History of Early Chemistry." *Jour. World History* 9: pp. 39–58.
DIEPGEN, PAUL. 1938. *Medizin und Kultur* (Stuttgart).
—— 1951. *Das Elixir: die Köstlichste der Arzneien* (Ingelheim am Rhein).
DUBS, HOMER H. 1947. "The Beginnings of Alchemy." *Isis* 38: pp. 62–86.
EASTON, STEWART C. 1952. *Roger Bacon and his Search for a Universal Science* (New York).
FORBES, R. J. 1948. *Short History of the Art of Distillation* (Leiden).
GANZENMÜLLER, W. ca. 1940. *L'Alchimie au moyen âge,* G. Petit-Dutaillis, tr. (Paris).
HOLMYARD, E. J. 1924. "Maslama al-Majriti and the *Rutbatu'l-Hakim.*" *Isis* 6: pp. 293–305.
—— 1957. *Alchemy* (Harmondsworth).
HOPKINS, ARTHUR JOHN. 1934. *Alchemy, Child of Greek Philosophy* (New York).
JOHNSON, OBED S. 1928. *A Study of Chinese Alchemy* (Shanghai).
KRAUS, PAUL. 1943. *Jabir ibn Hayyan: contribution à l'histoire des idées scientifiques dans l'Islam,* Mémoires présentés à l'Institut d'Égypte 44 (Cairo). 1: *Le Corpus des écrits Jabiriens;* 2: *Jabir et la science grecque.*
LEICESTER, HENRY M. 1956. *The Historical Background of Chemistry* (New York and London).
VON LIPPMANN, EDMUND O. 1919–1931; 1954. *Entstehung und Ausbreitung der Alchemie* (3 v., Berlin; Weinheim).
LITTLE, A. G., ed. 1914. *Roger Bacon Essays* (Oxford).
MULTHAUF, ROBERT P. 1954. "John of Rupescissa and the Origin of Medical Chemistry." *Isis* 45: pp. 359–367.
—— 1954. "Medical Chemistry and the 'Paracelsans.'" *Bull. Hist. of Medicine* 28: pp. 101–126.
—— 1956. "The Significance of Distillation in Renaissance Medical Chemistry." *Bull. Hist. of Medicine* 30: pp. 329–346.
NEEDHAM, JOSEPH. 1954 ff. See IV. and V. *b.*
PACHTER, HENRY M. 1951. *Magic into Science: the Story of Paracelsus* (New York).
PAGEL, WALTER. 1958. *Paracelsus: an Introduction to Philosophical Medicine in the Era of the Renaissance* (Basel and New York).

READ, JOHN. 1937. *Prelude to Chemistry: an Outline of Alchemy, its Literature and Relationships* (New York).
RUSKA, JULIUS. 1926. *Tabula Smaragdina: ein Beitrag zur Geschichte der hermetischen Literatur* (Heidelberg).
—— 1931. *Turba philosophorum: ein Beitrag zur Geschichte der Alchemie,* Quellen und Studien zur Geschichte der Naturwissenschaften und der Medizin 1 (Berlin).
—— 1935. "Die Alchemie ar-Razi's." *Der Islam* 22: pp. 281–319.
SINGER, DOROTHEA WALEY. 1932. "Alchemical Writings Attributed to Roger Bacon." *Speculum* 7: pp. 80–86.
SIVIN, NATHAN. 1965. "Preliminary Studies in Chinese Alchemy: The *Tan Ching Yao Chueh,* Attributed to Sun Ssu-mo." Doctoral thesis, Harvard U.
STAPLETON, HENRY ERNEST. 1905. "Sal Ammoniac: a Study in Primitive Chemistry." *Memoirs Asiatic Society of Bengal* (Calcutta) 1: pp. 25–41.
—— 1953. "The Antiquity of Alchemy." *Ambix* 5: pp. 1–43.
STAPLETON, HENRY ERNEST, and R. F. Azo. 1905. "Alchemical Equipment in the Eleventh Century, A.D." *Memoirs Asiatic Society of Bengal* (Calcutta) 1: pp. 47–71.
STAPLETON, HENRY ERNEST, and R. F. Azo. 1910. "An Alchemical Compilation of the Thirteenth Century, A.D." *Memoirs Asiatic Society of Bengal* (Calcutta) 3: pp. 57–94.
STAPLETON, HENRY ERNEST, R. F. Azo and M. HIDAYAT HUSAIN. 1927. "Chemistry in Iraq and Persia in the Tenth Century, A.D." *Memoirs Asiatic Society of Bengal* (Calcutta) 8: pp. 317–417.
TAYLOR, F. SHERWOOD. 1937. "The Origins of Greek Alchemy." *Ambix* 1: pp. 30–47.
—— 1949. *The Alchemists: Founders of Modern Chemistry,* Life of Science Library (New York).
—— 1953. "The Idea of the Quintessence." In Edgar A. Underwood, ed. *Science, Medicine, and History: Essays in Honour of Charles Singer* (2 v., London) 1: pp. 247–265.
TEMKIN, OWSEI. 1955. "Medicine and Graeco-Arabic Alchemy." *Bull. Hist. of Medicine* 29: pp. 134–153.
THORNDIKE, LYNN. 1923; 1934. *A History of Magic and Experimental Science* (New York) 2, 3, and 4.
WALEY, ARTHUR. 1930. "Notes on Chinese Alchemy." *Bull. School of Oriental Studies* (London) 6: pp. 1–24.
WELCH, HOLMES. 1956 and 1957. See IV. and V. *b.*
WILSON, WILLIAM JEROME. 1940. "Alchemy in China." *Ciba Symposia* 2: pp. 593–624.

VII. *a. The Hygienists: Primary Sources*

(CORNARO, LUIGI). Butler, William F., ed. 1903. *Discourses on the Temperate Life.* In *The Art of Living Long* (Milwaukee), pp. 37–114.
(HARVEY, WILLIAM). WILLIS, Robert, tr. 1847. "The Anatomical Examination of the Body of Thomas Parr." In *The Works of William Harvey* (London), pp. 587–592.
HUFELAND, CHRISTOPHER WILLIAM. 1797. *The Art of Prolonging Life* (2 v., London).
JACQUES, DANIEL HARRISON. 1859. *Physical Perfection: or, the Philosophy of Human Beauty; Showing how to Acquire and Retain Bodily Symmetry, Health and Vigor, Secure Long Life, and Avoid the Infirmities and Deformities of Age* (New York).
(LESSIUS, LEONARD). Smith, Timothy, tr. 1742. *Hygiasticon* (London).
SWEETSER, WILLIAM. 1867. *Human Life: Considered in its Present Condition and Future Developments, Especially with Reference to its Duration* (New York).
(TEMPLE, WILLIAM). 1770. "Of Health and Long Life." In *The Works of Sir William Temple* (London) 3: pp. 266–303.
THOMS, WILLIAM J. 1873. *Human Longevity, its Facts and its Fictions* (London).

VII. b. The Hygienists: Secondary Works

BURCKHARDT, JACOB. 1944. *The Civilization of the Renaissance*, S. G. C. Middlemore, tr. (London and New York).

BURSTEIN, SONA ROSA. 1955. See I. a. **10**: pp. 328–332.

DUBLIN, LOUIS I. 1952. "Longevity in Retrospect and Prospect." In Albert I. Lansing, ed. See I. b., pp. 203–220.

GRMEK, MIRKO D. 1958. See I. a.

GRUMAN, GERALD J. 1961. "The Rise and Fall of Prolongevity Hygiene: 1558–1873." *Bull. Hist. of Medicine* **35**: pp. 221–229.

MARONCELLI, PIERO. 1842. "Biography of Alvise [Luigi] Cornaro." In John Burdell, ed. *The Discourses and Letters of Louis Cornaro, On a Sober and Temperate Life* (New York), pp. 127–153.

ROSEN, GEORGE. 1958. *A History of Public Health* (New York).

SHRYOCK, RICHARD H. 1947. See VIII. b.

SIGERIST, HENRY E. 1956. *Landmarks in the History of Hygiene* (London).

WALKER, WILLIAM B. 1954. "Luigi Cornaro, a Renaissance Writer on Personal Hygiene." *Bull. Hist. of Medicine* **28**: pp. 525–534.

ZEMAN, FREDERIC D. 1942–1950. See I. a. **12**: pp. 833–846, 939–953 and **17**: pp. 53–68.

VIII. a. The Philosophes: Primary Sources

(BACON, FRANCIS). Rawley, William, tr. 1638. *History, Naturall and Experimentall, of Life and Death* (London).

(——). Spedding, James, Robert Leslie Ellis, and Douglas Denon Heath, eds. 1861 ff. *Works* (15 v., Boston).

(CABANIS, PIERRE J. G.). Lehec, Claude, and Jean Cazeneuve, eds. 1956. *Œuvres philosophiques*, Corpus général des philosophes français (2 v., Paris).

(DE CONDORCET, ANTOINE-NICOLAS). Barraclough, June, tr. 1955. *Sketch for a Historical Picture of the Progress of the Human Mind*, Library of Ideas (New York).

(——). O'Connor, A. Condorcet, and M. F. Arago, eds. 1847–1849. *Œuvres* (12 v., Paris).

(DESCARTES, RENÉ). Adam, Charles, and Paul Tannery, eds. 1897–1909. *Œuvres* (11 v., Paris).

(——). Roth, Leon, ed. 1926. *Correspondence of Descartes and Constantyn Huygens: 1635–1647* (Oxford).

(——). Veitch, John, tr. 1912. *A Discourse on Method, etc.*, Everyman's Library (London, Toronto and New York).

(FRANKLIN, BENJAMIN). Cohen, I. Bernard, ed. 1941. *Benjamin Franklin's Experiments: a New Edition of Franklin's Experiments and Observations on Electricity* (Cambridge, Mass.).

(——). Cohen, I. Bernard, ed. 1954. *Some Account of the Pennsylvania Hospital* (Baltimore).

(——). Farrand, Max, ed. 1949. *Benjamin Franklin's Memoirs: Parallel Text Edition* (Berkeley, Calif.).

(——). Labaree, Leonard W., and Whitfield J. Bell, Jr., eds. 1959 ff. *The Papers of Benjamin Franklin* (New Haven, Conn.).

(——). Smyth, Albert H., ed. 1905–1907. *Writings* (10 v., New York).

(GODWIN, WILLIAM). Priestley, F. E. L., ed. 1946. *Enquiry Concerning Political Justice, and its Influence on Morals and Happiness*, third edition with variant readings of the first and second (3 v., Toronto).

HUNTER, JOHN. 1841. *Lectures on the Principles of Surgery* (Philadelphia).

MALTHUS, THOMAS ROBERT. 1798. *An Essay on the Principle of Population, as it Affects the Future Improvement of Society, with Remarks on the Speculations of Mr. Godwin, M. Condorcet, and Other Writers* (London).

PRICE, RICHARD. 1787. *The Evidence for a Future Period of Improvement in the State of Mankind, with the Means and Duty of Promoting it* (London).

PRIESTLEY, JOSEPH. 1806. *Memoirs, with a Continuation by his Son and Observations by Thomas Cooper and Reverend William Christie* (Northumberland, Pa.).

(Progress, ideas of). Teggart, Frederick J., and George H. Hildebrand, eds. 1949. *The Idea of Progress: a Collection of Readings* (Berkeley and Los Angeles).

(Royal Society). Lowthorp, John, ed. 1716. *The Philosophical Transactions and Collections to the End of the Year 1700, Abridg'd and Dispos'd under General Heads* (2nd ed., London) **3**.

(ZAMBECCARI, JOSEPH). 1941. Saul Jarcho, tr. "Experiments Concerning the Excision of Various Organs from Living Animals." *Bull. Hist. of Medicine* **9**: pp. 311–331.

VIII. b. The Philosophes: Secondary Works

ACKERKNECHT, ERWIN H. 1955. *A Short History of Medicine* (New York).

ADAM, CHARLES. 1910. *Vie et œuvres de Descartes: étude historique* (Paris).

BAILLET, ADRIEN. 1691. *La Vie de Descartes* (2 v., Paris).

BAILLIE, JOHN. 1950. *The Belief in Progress* (London).

BECKER, CARL L. 1932. *The Heavenly City of the Eighteenth-Century Philosophers* (New Haven).

—— 1935. *Everyman His Own Historian* (New York).

—— 1946. *Benjamin Franklin: a Biographical Sketch* (Ithaca).

BERDYAEV, NICHOLAS. 1936. *The Meaning of History* (London).

BERTHIER, AUGUSTE GEORGES. 1914; 1920. "Le Mécanisme cartésien et la physiologie au XVIIe siècle." *Isis* **2**: pp. 37–89; **3**: pp. 21–58.

BILLINGTON, JAMES H. 1960. "The Intelligentsia and the Religion of Humanity." *Amer. Hist. Review* **65**: pp. 807–821.

BRAILSFORD, H. N. 1913. *Shelley, Godwin and Their Circle* (London).

BRINTON, CRANE. 1930. *The Jacobins: an Essay in the New History* (New York).

—— 1959. *A History of Western Morals* (New York).

—— 1963. *Ideas and Men* (2nd ed., Englewood Cliffs, N. J.).

BROWN, HARCOURT. 1936. "The Utilitarian Motive in the Age of Descartes." *Annals of Science* **1**: pp. 182–192.

—— 1948. "Jean Denis and Transfusion of Blood: Paris, 1667–1668." *Isis* **39**: pp. 15–29.

BURY, J. B. 1932. *The Idea of Progress* (New York).

CHORON, JACQUES. 1964. See I. b.

COHEN, I. BERNARD. 1953. *Benjamin Franklin: his Contribution to the American Tradition* (Indianapolis).

—— 1956. *Franklin and Newton: an Inquiry into Speculative Newtonian Experimental Science and Franklin's Work in Electricity as an Example Thereof*, Mem. Amer. Philos. Soc. **43** (Philadelphia).

DEBUS, ALLEN G. 1964. "The Paracelsian Aerial Niter." *Isis* **55**: pp. 43–61.

DELVAILLE, JULES. 1910. *Essai sur l'histoire de l'idée de progrès, jusqu'à la fin du XVIIIe siècle*, Collection historique des grands philosophes (Paris).

DES MAIZEAUX, P., ed. and tr. 1728. *The Works of St. Evremond, with the Life of the Author by Des Maizeaux* (2nd ed., London) **1**.

DILLER, THEODORE. 1912. *Franklin's Contribution to Medicine* (Brooklyn).

DREYFUS-LE FOYER, H. 1937. "Les Conceptions médicales de Descartes." *Revue de métaphysique et de morale* **44**: pp. 237–286.

DUBOS, RENÉ. 1961. *The Dreams of Reason: Science and Utopias* (New York).

EISELEY, LOREN. 1962. *Francis Bacon and the Modern Dilemma* (Lincoln, Nebr.).

ETTINGER, ROBERT C. W. 1964. *The Prospect of Immortality* (New York).

—— 1965. "The Frozen Christian." *Christian Century* **82**: pp. 1313–1315.

——1966. "Science and Immortality." *Yale Scientific Magazine* **40**, 7 : pp. 5–8, 20.

FARRINGTON, BENJAMIN. 1951. *Francis Bacon: Philosopher of Industrial Science* (London).

FAY, BERNARD. 1929. *Franklin, the Apostle of Modern Times* (Boston).

FLEISHER, DAVID. 1951. *William Godwin: a Study in Liberalism* (London).

FOSTER, MICHAEL. 1901. *Lectures on the History of Physiology During the Sixteenth, Seventeenth and Eighteenth Centuries* (Cambridge).

GAY, PETER. 1964. *The Party of Humanity* (New York).

GRUMAN, GERALD J. 1956. "C. A. Stephens: Popular Author and Prophet of Gerontology." *New England Jour. Medicine* **254**: pp. 658–660.

—— 1959. "C. A. Stephens: a Pioneer of American Gerontology." *Geriatrics* **14**: pp. 332–336.

HALDANE, ELIZABETH S. 1905. *Descartes, his Life and Times* (London).

HALE, EDWARD E., and EDWARD E. HALE, JR. 1888. *Franklin in France* (2 v., Boston).

KEILIN, D. 1959. "The Problem of Anabiosis or Latent Life: History and Current Concept." *Proceedings Royal Society* B **150**: pp. 149–191.

(Life Extension Society). 1964 ff. *Newsletter* (Washington).

MAHAFFY, J. P. 1902. *Descartes,* Philosophical Classics for English Readers (Edinburgh and London).

MALUF, N. S. R. 1954. "History of Blood Transfusion." *Jour. Hist. of Medicine* **9**: pp. 59–107.

MANUEL, FRANK E. 1962. *The Prophets of Paris* (Cambridge, Mass.).

MARITAIN, JACQUES. 1944. *The Dream of Descartes, Together with Some Other Essays.* Mabelle L. Andison, tr. (New York).

MARTIN, KINGSLEY. 1962; 1963. *French Liberal Thought in the Eighteenth Century* (3rd ed., London; New York).

NEUBURGER, MAX. 1926. "Lord Bacon's Relations to Medicine." *Medical Life* **33**: pp. 149–169.

PARKES, A. S. 1955. "Preservation of Tissue *in vitro* for the Study of Ageing." In G. E. W. Wolstenholme and Cecilia M. O'Connor, eds., *General Aspects of Ageing,* Ciba Foundation Colloquia on Ageing **1** (Boston), pp. 162–169.

PAUL, C. KEGAN. 1876. *William Godwin: his Friends and Contemporaries* (2 v., London).

PEPPER, WILLIAM. 1911. *The Medical Side of Benjamin Franklin* (Philadelphia).

ROCKWOOD, RAYMOND O., ed. 1958. *Carl Becker's Heavenly City Revisited* (Ithaca, N. Y.).

SAMPSON, R. V. 1956. *Progress in the Age of Reason: the Seventeenth Century to the Present Day* (Cambridge, Mass.).

SCHAPIRO, J. SALWYN. 1934. *Condorcet and the Rise of Liberalism* (New York).

SHRYOCK, RICHARD H. 1936. *The Development of Modern Medicine: an Interpretation of the Social and Scientific Factors Involved* (Philadelphia and London).

—— 1956. "The Significance of Medicine in American History." *Amer. Historical Review* **62**: pp. 81–91.

SMITH, NORMAN KEMP. 1952. *New Studies in the Philosophy of Descartes: Descartes as Pioneer* (London).

SPEDDING, JAMES. 1878. *An Account of the Life and Times of Francis Bacon* (2 v., Boston).

STEPHENS, C. A. 1903. *Natural Salvation: the Message of Science* (Norway Lake, Maine).

THOMSON, ELIZABETH H. 1963. "The Role of Physicians in the Humane Societies of the Eighteenth Century." *Bull. History of Medicine* **37**: pp. 43–51.

VAN DOREN, CARL. 1938. *Benjamin Franklin* (New York).

VARTANIAN, ARAM. 1953. *Diderot and Descartes: a Study of Scientific Naturalism in the Enlightenment,* History of Ideas Series **6** (Princeton).

ZIMMERMAN, LEO M., and KATHERINE M. HOWELL. 1932. "History of Blood Transfusion." *Annals Medical History* **4**: pp. 415–433.

THE LITERATURE OF
DEATH AND DYING

Abrahamsson, Hans. **The Origin of Death:** Studies in African Mythology. 1951

Alden, Timothy. **A Collection of American Epitaphs and Inscriptions with Occasional Notes.** Five vols. in two. 1814

Austin, Mary. **Experiences Facing Death.** 1931

Bacon, Francis. **The Historie of Life and Death with Observations Naturall and Experimentall for the Prolongation of Life.** 1638

Barth, Karl. **The Resurrection of the Dead.** 1933

Bataille, Georges. **Death and Sensuality:** A Study of Eroticism and the Taboo. 1962

Bichat, [Marie François] Xavier. **Physiological Researches on Life and Death.** 1827

Browne, Thomas. **Hydriotaphia.** 1927

Carrington, Hereward. **Death:** Its Causes and Phenomena with Special Reference to Immortality. 1921

Comper, Frances M. M., editor. **The Book of the Craft of Dying and Other Early English Tracts Concerning Death.** 1917

Death and the Visual Arts. 1976

Death as a Speculative Theme in Religious, Scientific, and Social Thought. 1976

Donne, John. **Biathanatos.** 1930

Farber, Maurice L. **Theory of Suicide.** 1968

Fechner, Gustav Theodor. **The Little Book of Life After Death.** 1904

Frazer, James George. **The Fear of the Dead in Primitive Religion.** Three vols. in one. 1933/1934/1936

Fulton, Robert. **A Bibliography on Death, Grief and Bereavement:** 1845-1975. 1976

Gorer, Geoffrey. **Death, Grief, and Mourning.** 1965

Gruman, Gerald J. **A History of Ideas About the Prolongation of Life.** 1966

Henry, Andrew F. and James F. Short, Jr. **Suicide and Homicide.** 1954

Howells, W[illiam] D[ean], et al. **In After Days;** Thoughts on the Future Life. 1910

Irion, Paul E. **The Funeral:** Vestige or Value? 1966

Landsberg, Paul-Louis. **The Experience of Death:** The Moral Problem of Suicide. 1953

Maeterlinck, Maurice. **Before the Great Silence.** 1937

Maeterlinck, Maurice. **Death.** 1912

Metchnikoff, Élie. **The Nature of Man:** Studies in Optimistic Philosophy. 1910

Metchnikoff, Élie. **The Prolongation of Life:** Optimistic Studies. 1908

Munk, William. **Euthanasia.** 1887

Osler, William. **Science and Immortality.** 1904

Return to Life: Two Imaginings of the Lazarus Theme. 1976

Stephens, C[harles] A[sbury]. **Natural Salvation:** The Message of Science. 1905

Sulzberger, Cyrus. **My Brother Death.** 1961

Taylor, Jeremy. **The Rule and Exercises of Holy Dying.** 1819

Walker, G[eorge] A[lfred]. **Gatherings from Graveyards.** 1839

Warthin, Aldred Scott. **The Physician of the Dance of Death.** 1931

Whiter, Walter. **Dissertation on the Disorder of Death.** 1819

Whyte, Florence. **The Dance of Death in Spain and Catalonia.** 1931

Wolfenstein, Martha. **Disaster:** A Psychological Essay. 1957

Worcester, Alfred. **The Care of the Aged, the Dying, and the Dead.** 1950

Zandee, J[an]. **Death as an Enemy According to Ancient Egyptian Conceptions.** 1960

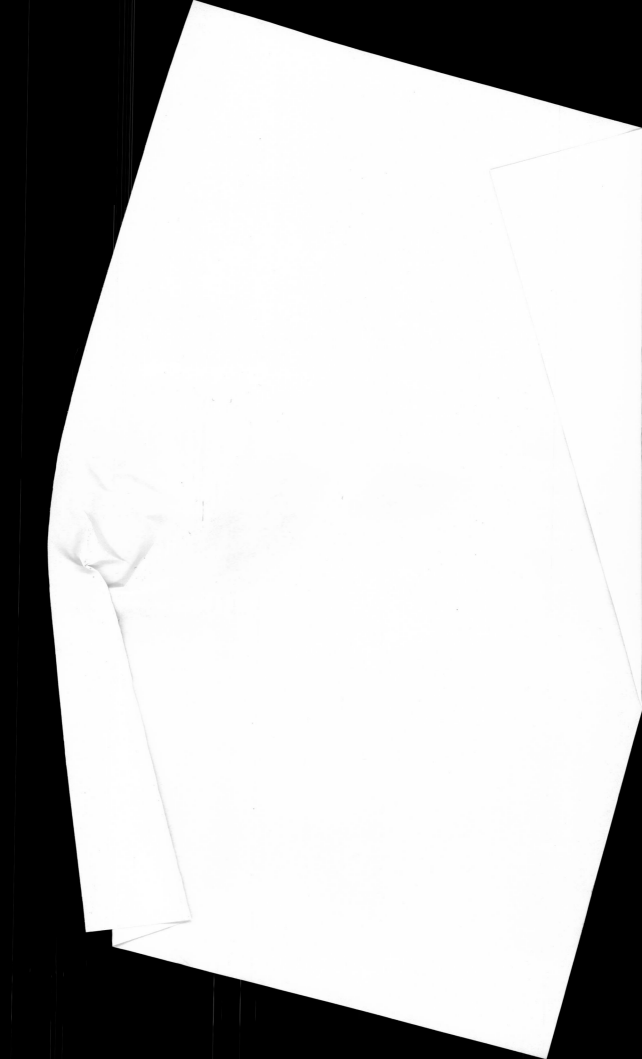

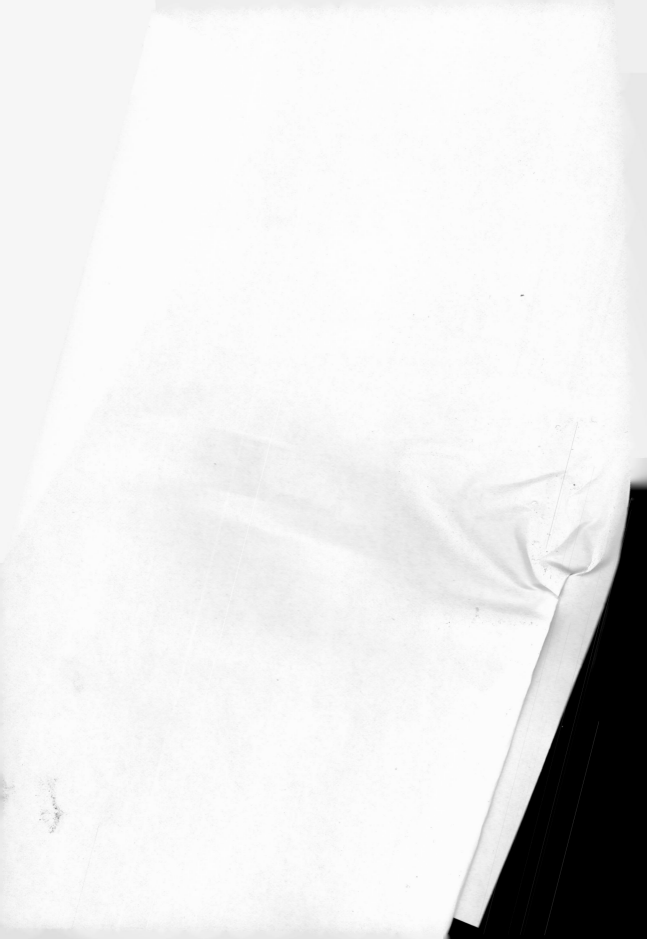